When to Bypass Back Surgery

JOSE H. AUDAY is a medical doctor.

Board Certified by the American Board of Orthopaedic Surgery
Emeritus Fellow of the American Academy of Orthopaedic Surgeons
Fellow of the American College of Surgeons
Emeritus Member of the Arthroscopy Association of North America
Emeritus Member of the International Society of Arthroscopy, Knee Surgery and
    Orthopaedic Sports Medicine
Former Faculty Member of Hahnemann Medical College of Philadelphia
Former Attending Surgeon at Hahnemann Hospital, Philadelphia
Former Chief Orthopaedic Surgery at Jefferson Park Hospital, Philadelphia
Former Acting-Chief at Albert Einstein Medical Center (Southern Division),
    Philadelphia
Former Attending Orthopaedic Surgeon at St. Agnes Hospital, Philadelphia
Former Attending Surgeon at St. Mary's Hospital, Philadelphia
Former Attending Senior Surgeon at St. Joseph's Hospital, Philadelphia

When to Bypass Back Surgery

Jose H. Auday, M.D., F.A.C.S.

To order additional copies of this book, contact:
Xlibris Corporation
1-888-795-4274
www.Xlibris.com
Orders@Xlibris.com
51534

Contents

TO MY FIVE SONS:

Chomie,

David,

Paul,

Robert, and

Joseph.

Acknowledgment

I am grateful to Dr. Diana Goldman for giving me encouragement, for reviewing, correcting, and giving me valuable personal knowledge in the writing of this book.

Introduction

Back pain is one of the most common physical conditions affecting humans.

Low back pain is one of the most prevalent and costly health problems in the industrialized world. Approximately 80% of United States population report having had low back pain at some point in their lives, resulting in more lost productivity than any other medical condition. Although its frequency is so high, it is still difficult to choose between surgical and medical treatment.

"The literature comparing the efficacy of surgical and medical treatment for low back pain is limited. Not surprisingly, the use of surgery for low back pain varies widely across the United States. To establish clinical consensus, we need better evidence about the efficacy of surgery" (Effective Clinical Practice, Sept./Oct. 1999, Medical vs. Surgical treatment for low back pain: Evidence and Clinical, Nancy J. O. Burkmeyer, James Weinstein, MD).

"In the United States alone, the annual combined cost of back pain and related disability compensation is estimated at fifty billion dollars" ("Low-Back Pain," *Scientific American*, Vol. 279, August, 48-53, 1998).

"Low back pain is a costly and often seriously disabling condition that affect industries in all countries. Low back injuries are a major industrial cause of disability in the United States, with 2% of the workforce incurring back injuries each year. Back injuries are the most expensive healthcare problem for the thirty- to fifty-year-old group and are the leading cause of disability in the United States for persons younger than forty-five years" (Timothy R. Dillingham, MD, MS, JAMA.1998; 279:1826-1828).

"In the US, several studies suggest that approximately 25% of adults report having had low back pain in the past three months, whereas 7.6%

report at least one episode of severe acute low back pain within the previous year. Clinical evidence suggests that regardless of treatment, most low back pain improves within one month. Available treatment options run from watchful waiting to conservative treatment with pharmacological and nonpharmacologic modalities to invasive procedures such as spinal surgery" (Medscape, Guidelines Issued Management of Low Back Pain CMS/CE, Laurie Barclay, MD, Oct. 2,2007).

Backache is caused by mechanical conditions related to biped stance (erect position, walking upright) of the *Homo sapiens.* Biped stance gives us the advantage of using the upper extremities (arms, hands), but make the erect spine more vulnerable to the force of gravity.

One-third of sedentary workers and nearly half of the workers in heavy industry will incur a significant episode of low back pain.

Risk factors involved in this condition could be age, weight, heavy lifting, and prolonged sitting position (truck drivers), etc.

Low back pain (LBP) is the number one compensable work-related injury and the most common cause of absence from work.

"In 2005 there were 1,175,000 inpatient spinal surgeries in the USA alone, according to market research from Spinemarket and Newsletter Orthopedic Network News" (FORTUNE, Sept. 4, 2006, Pg. 104).

The proposal of this book is to discuss diagnosis and treatment of what we call mechanical low back pain, which as I already mentioned, is one of the most frequent medical conditions found in our society.

People should know that low back pain could be also due to nonmechanical causes, which should be diagnosed and treated by a physician.

Let's enumerate the most common of these conditions (due to nonmechanical causes):

1. **Inflammatory and metabolic in origin**

   a. Ankylosis spondylitis—A disease due to abnormal bony union (calcification) of all the ligaments of the spine, also known as "bamboo spine"
   b. Psoriasis—Chronic inflammatory skin disease capable to involve joints
   c. Inflammatory bowel disease
   d. Reiter's syndrome—Disease in man

e. Osteoporosis—Loss of bony mass, with fractures.
f. Osteomalacia—Weak bones, with frequent fractures, due to lack of Vitamin D (rare in USA)
g. Paget's disease—Abnormal absorption and reabsorption of bone, in a chaotic manner
h. Hyperparathyroidism—Excessive production of parathohormone
i. Hyperthyroidism—Excessive production of thyroid hormone
j. Cushing's syndrome—Excessive production of suprarenal hormone
k. Fibromyalgia—Generalized weakness and muscle ache, of unknown etiology; it used to be called fibrositis, perhaps a neurological condition not helped by nonsteroidal analgesic drugs; not everybody believes in this condition, including the author.

2. Tumors

a. Primary—Of the spinal cord or skeletal, benign like neuroma or an osteoma, malignant like osteosarcoma
b. Metastatic—Disseminated from another region of the body, like breast in woman and prostate in man
c. Tumor and "like tumors"—Related to blood organs, like plasma cell tumor, multiple myeloma, and lymphoma

3. Infections

a. Septicemia—Grave febrile condition due to bacteremia (generalized spread of germs through the blood)
b. Osteomyelitis—Localized or focal bone infection
c. Discitis—Infection of the intervertebral disc, usually seen as a postsurgical complication
d. Epidural abscess—Localized infection of the duramater (one of the layers of the meninges, membrane surrounding the central nervous system)
e. Tuberculosis
g. Brucellosis—Infection due to bacteria, causing undulant fever, transmitted to humans by goats, etc. (rare in USA)

4. **Pain referred from another area of the body**

    a. Pelvic and gynecological—Like a retroverted uterus
    b. Gastrointestinal conditions—Like gastric ulcer, adherent to lumbar spine
    c. Renal—Related to the kidney, like a renal colic
    d. Aneurysm—Localized enlargement or occlusion of the abdominal aorta
    e. Pancreas—Chronic pancreatitis like seen in alcoholism
    f. Retroperitoneal conditions—Behind abdominal cavity, like adenopathies (enlarged lymph nodes)
    g. Hip disease—Arthritis or arthrosis of this joint

In order to understand the complex and real enigma of low back pain, I will summarize the anatomy and physiology of the lumbar region, the bony and soft tissue parts (muscles, tendons, and ligaments).

I will divide low back pain according to age—childhood, adulthood, and elderhood—since in each of these periods it requires a different medical approach and treatment.

Chapter 1

Anatomy

The spinal column is designed for many purposes. It is, in the first place, a sustaining rod which is implanted into the pelvic rim and maintains the body in upright position; it carries the thoracic cage and sustains the balance between it and the abdominal cavity; it serves as a post of anchorage for many powerful muscles which maintain the balance of the spine and perform all spinal movement; and it furnishes the site of origin for many muscles of the shoulder and pelvic girdle. The spinal cord is encased in the vertebral column and protected against mechanical injuries (Kinesiology of the Human Body, Arthur Steindler, Pub. Thomas).

The spinal cord is protected by surrounding fluid enclosed in a large pouch, the meninges (fig.1). This is a tough membranous-like tube, which runs from base of the skull to first or second sacral segment and keeps the cord and "horse tail" (cauda equina) buffered in a fluid medium.

Membranes Meninge

Severed Meninge
View From Behind

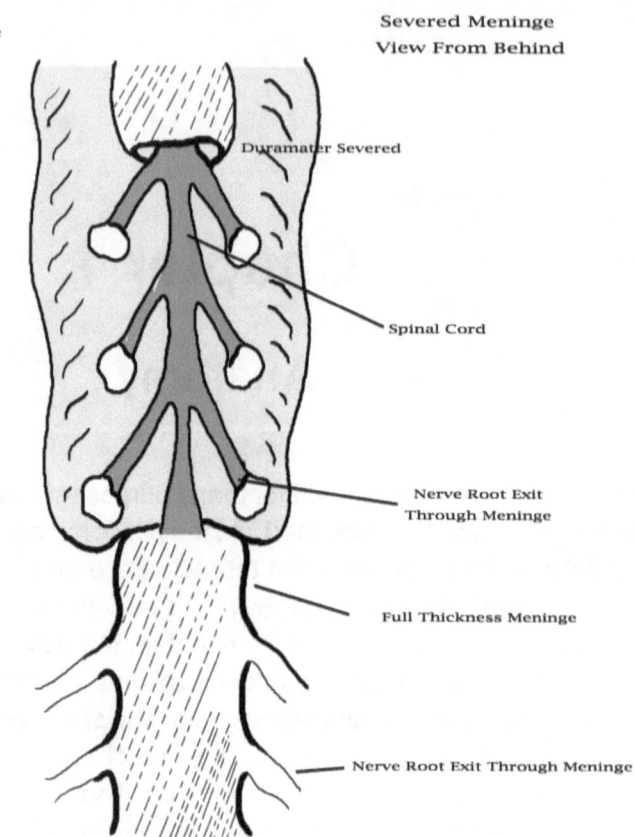

Duramater Severed

Spinal Cord

Nerve Root Exit
Through Meninge

Full Thickness Meninge

Nerve Root Exit Through Meninge

Cut Through Upper Lumbar Vertebra

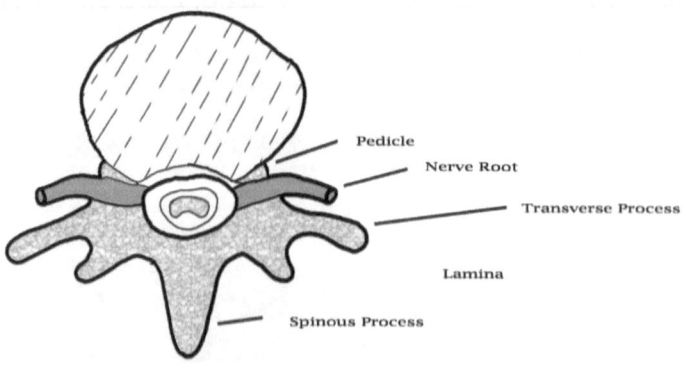

Pedicle

Nerve Root

Transverse Process

Lamina

Spinous Process

Fig. 1

These elements are inside a long bony canal, the spine, composed by superimposed number of links movable against each other. The vertebral bodies are held together by ligamentous and muscular structures. From head down, there are seven cervical vertebrae, twelve dorsal vertebrae (back of rib cage), five lumbar vertebrae, the sacrum (the five fused vertebrae which is implanted into the pelvis and forms part of the pelvic ring), and the three or four coccygeal segments, remaining of the tail of animals (fig. 2).

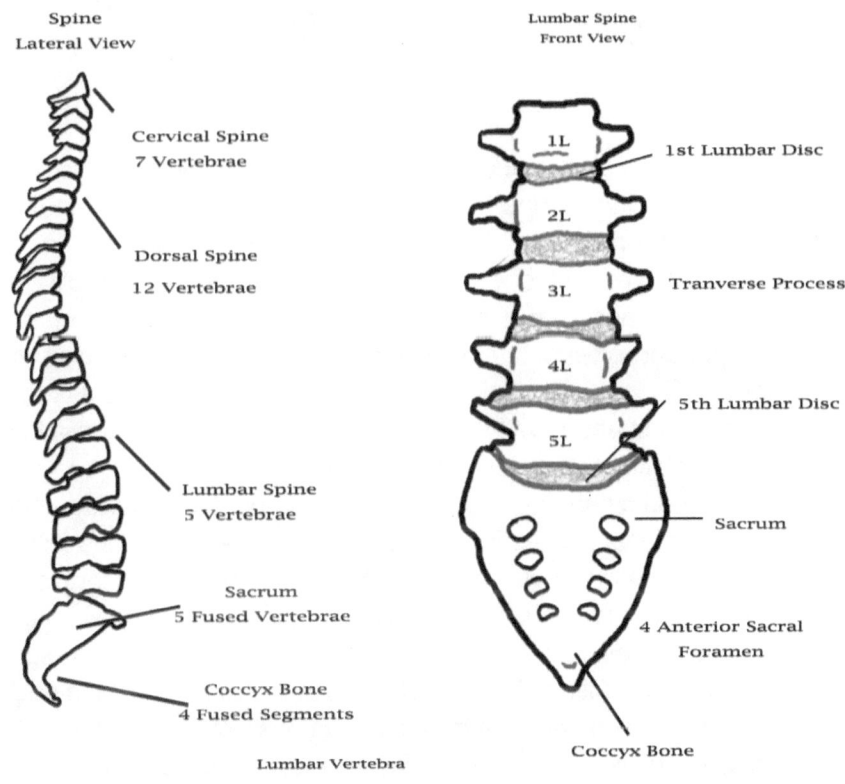

Fig. 2

Lower back pain is related to the so-called lumbosacral region.

The spinal cord ends at the level of the second lumbar vertebrae, and it continues by the cauda equina (like horse tail), which are the nerve roots carrying the impulses to make move or feel your lower extremities, bringing sensations to touch, heat, cold, and pain.

Then the cord and the horsetail are protected by the spinal canal, formed by joint—superimposed vertebrae (fig.3).

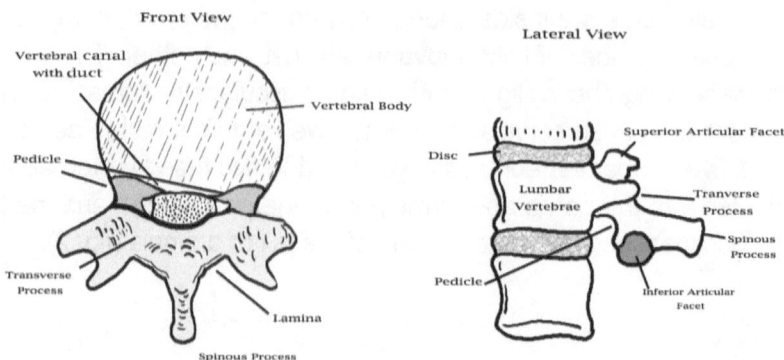

Fig. 3

A vertebra has a body and an arch, joined together by the pedicles. The so-called neural arch carries three apophyseal processes: the articular, (superior and inferior facets), the transverse, and the spinous.

Body-to-body are joint together by a disc (a soft tissue structure, which works like a shock absorber, like a cushion between vertebrae). The disc is the most important soft structure of the functional spine. It is in the disc where the center of motion lies, and all motion between vertebrae are associated with adaptational changes within the disc itself. This is made possible only because of its elastic properties, which permit the disc to change in shape. The disc is formed by an outer fibrocartilaginous ring, the so-called annulus fibrosus. The center of the disc is occupied by the so-called nucleus pulposus (fig. 4), a gelatinous mass, elastic, and capable of changing its form as well as its position within the ring. Tilting motions of the vertebral bodies against each other produce asymmetrical compression of the disc; the disc responds by changing its form. Tilting of the vertebral bodies usually forces the nucleus pulposus toward the convexity of the curve. For example, bending your back forward push the nucleus pulposus backward, making it to herniate posteriorly (herniated lumbar disc). In all these joints the facets glide upon each other during motion. Therefore, one must look for the center of motion somewhere else; this center is the intervertebral disc.

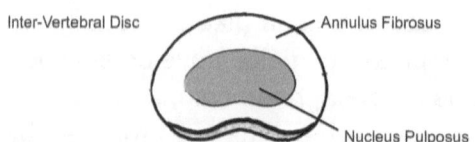

Fig. 4

It represents a universal joint, which allows rotary motion in the three planes: flexion and extension in the sagittal, side bending to right and left in the frontal, and rotation to right and left in the transverse plane.

Finally, the disc is under constant compression in the upright position (orthograde position); as a matter of fact, you are taller in recumbency, especially after a night's rest. The arch encircles the cord and forms the tunnel. Each arch joins the above and below arch by small joints called superior and inferior facets (the articular, apophyseal process); the back part of the arch ends in what we call spinous process (tip of bones seen and palpable on the middle or center of your back).

Between each bone arch, a small ovoid tunnel is formed called foramen. It is the small conduit where the right and left nerve roots exit the spine (fig.5).

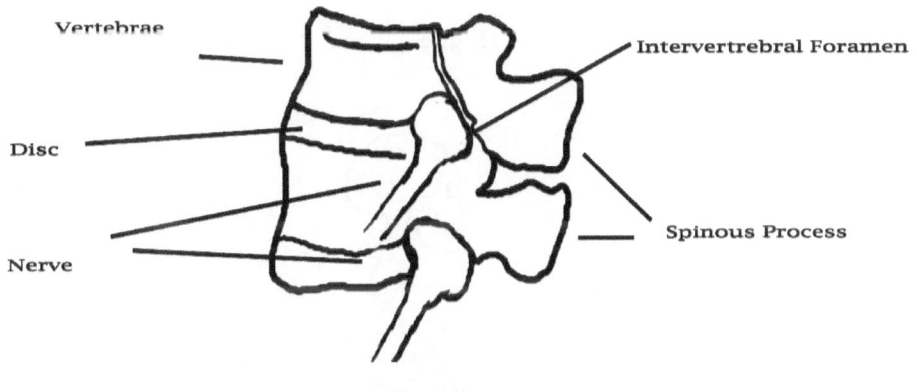

Vertebrae

Intervertrebral Foramen

Disc

Spinous Process

Nerve

Fig. 5

The vertebrae are held together by ligaments and muscles, restraining motion to the vertebra and preserving stability.

The ligaments (like cords) extend from one spinous process to the other above and below of the superior and inferior vertebra, so from the facets and vertebral bodies (fig. 6). We have short and long muscles; the short do extend from one vertebra to the above and below vertebra; the long muscles do extend along the entire lumbosacral region; these powerful muscles start and end by flat type of cord tissue into the bone called insertion points (fig. 7).

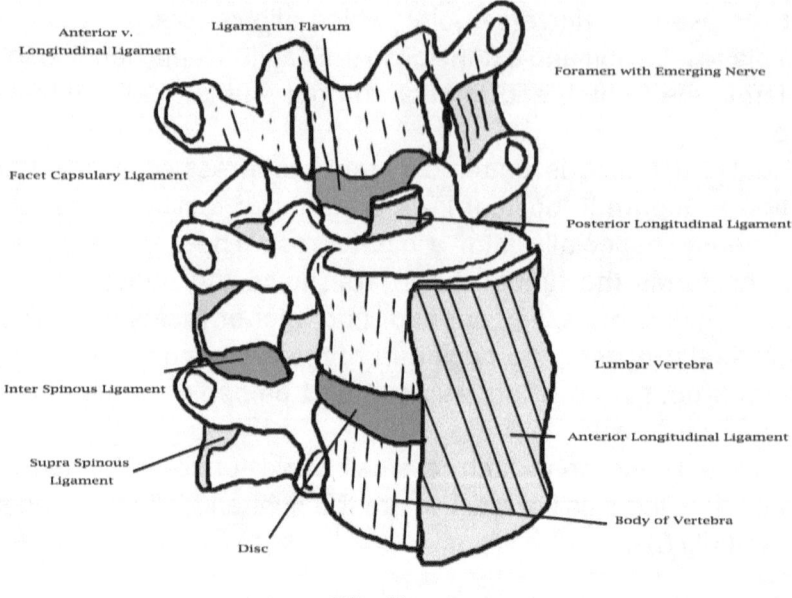

Oblique View

Fig. 6

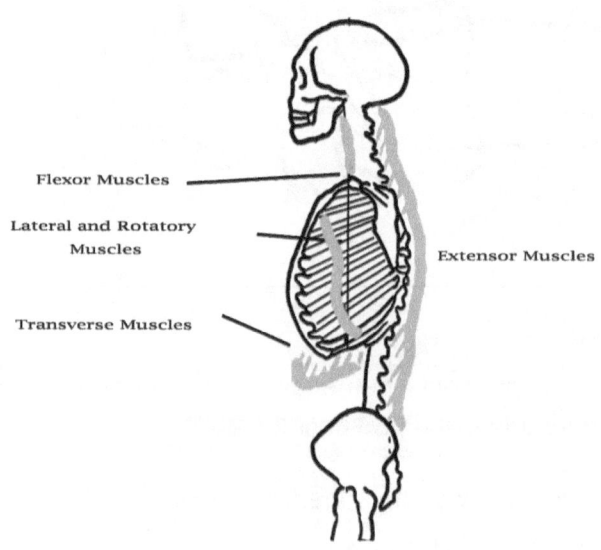

Fig. 7

There are four muscles systems in the lumbosacral region:

1. Extensors of the lumbar spine (backward motion)—the sacrospinalis system (erector spinae, sacrolumbaris, and longissimus dorsi)

2. Flexors of the lumbar spine (forward bending)—rectus abdominis, external and internal obliques, and the spinofemoral muscles, which flexes trunk against thigh when the later is fixed (iliacus and psoas muscles)
3. Lateral benders of the lumbar spine (bending to right and left)—external and internal obliques, quadratus lumbaris, and transversus abdominis.
4. Rotator of the lumbar spine (turning right and left)—external and internal obliques.

The spine extends from the base of the skull to the sacrococcygeal region as already explained, seeing from the back (we can not see it from the front, except on an X-ray). In this view the spine is vertical (frontal plane) (see fig. 2), but seeing from the side (sagittal plane) has several "curvatures" (fig. 8), an upper curvature with the concavity looking backward, so-called cervical lordosis, followed by the opposite, a curvature with the convexity looking backward "dorsal khyphosis," followed by the opposite a curvature with the concavity looking backward "lumbar lordosis." These curvatures are somewhat elastic and work like shock absorbers by increasing or decreasing its curvatures instead of being a vertical pillar. It is interesting to notice that in the lumbar region the articulations of the vertebrae first, second, third, and fourth are aligned more in the sagittal plane. This arrangement provides for more axial rotation and forward and backward motion (flexion-extension) and little side motion. Side motion, bending to right and left is taken by the sacrolumbar articulations (joints), which are arranged in the frontal plane.

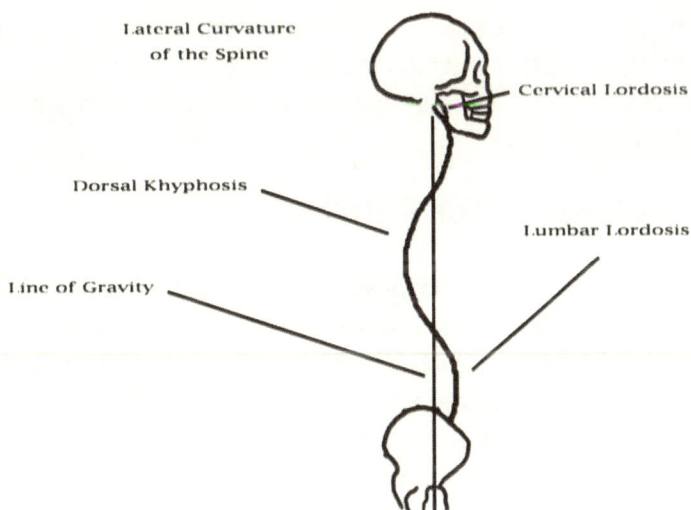

Lateral Curvature of the Spine

Cervical Lordosis

Dorsal Khyphosis

Lumbar Lordosis

Line of Gravity

Fig. 8

So the complex motion of the spine in one way or another makes the spine more vulnerable to get hurt. For better understanding, the reader could visualize that the spine moves in the three planes of the space:

1. In the frontal plane: bends right and left
2. In the sagittal plane: bends forward and backward
3. In the transversal plane: rotates to the right and left

A lot has been written about the mechanics of the spine, the bipodal or erect position of the *Homo sapiens*, and its relation to low back pain

The whole body weight is transmitted from the lumbosacral region (back) to both lower extremities, being the center of gravity around the second lumbar vertebra. Quoting James Cyriax (Textbook of Orthopaedic Medicine, volume 1, 6th edition, Baillieri-Tindal), "Why does ordinary use of the joints of the spine cause pain so readily, when the other joints of the body can so often withstand lifelong exertion without causing trouble? The answer is man's acquisition of the erect posture. Recent discoveries in Africa suggest that men walked upright there between three and five million years ago, long enough, one might have thought, to allow better adaptation. But the cerebellum has caught the vertebral column unprepared, the capacity to maintain equilibrium on two legs outstripping the evolution of the spine. As soon as man learned to stand, the function of the spine altered; hence the whole column should have been redesigned."

Quadrupeds walking on four legs seem to suffer, in lesser degree, of back pain. There was an old German treatment for scoliosis (abnormal curvatures of the spine) in which the patient with scoliosis was put on an exercise program consisting in walking with the legs and arms imitating a quadruped gait.

Why Do We Get Back Pain?

Back pain is a complex condition, Where does the pain originate? From the vertebral bone? From the disc? From the Intervertebral joints? From the ligaments? From the muscles? Or the nerve roots? The answer is YES! It could come from any of these structures, making the prognosis and the treatment somewhat different. Recent studies tend to support the idea that most cases of low back pain are caused by disc or facet damage.

Classification of Low Back Pain:

I will use different terms to describe certain types of pain, as follows:

1. Low backache—I will describe as mild discomfort.
2. Low back pain—Sharp back pain of different intensity.
3. Lumbago—A sudden attack of sharp back pain with temporary "fixing" of your spine.
4. Sciatica—A sharp pain that runs along the sciatic nerve pathway through the buttock and radiates down the back of the thigh and leg into the foot

Chapter 2

Children Low Back Pain

I separate this condition in children from adults because diagnosis, prognosis, and treatment could be different. Any low back pain in a child, over a week duration (except trauma), should take a parent to seek medical advice. Children are very honest and do not fake about pain. Localized pain, progressive, or at rest should be of more concern to parents. Sometimes the child will finger-point to the painful area. Night pain and to be awaken by pain would point to an inflammatory or tumor condition.

The following are common causes of low back pain in children, some could be congenital (from birth) and others developmental:

1. Spondylolisis—A congenital anomaly that could advance to spondylolisthesis as the child grows up. Normally, the posterior arch gets fused to the vertebral body. However, when for unknown reason this does not happen, the gap between the body and the arch is called spondylolisis (fig. 9). If the posterior arch or the body slips, it becomes a spondylolisthesis (fig. 10). The most common anomaly is found in the fifth lumbar vertebra. As a result of this mechanical anomaly, the child will complain of pain aggravated by bending, pushing, or lifting, and some can even develop leg pain (radiculitis). This condition requires close orthopedic care.

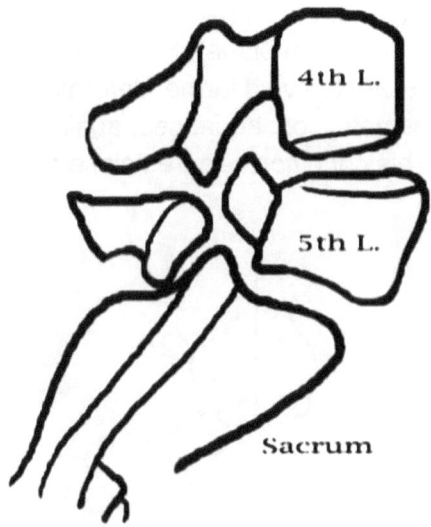

Spondylolysis 5th Lumbar Vertebrae

Fig. 9

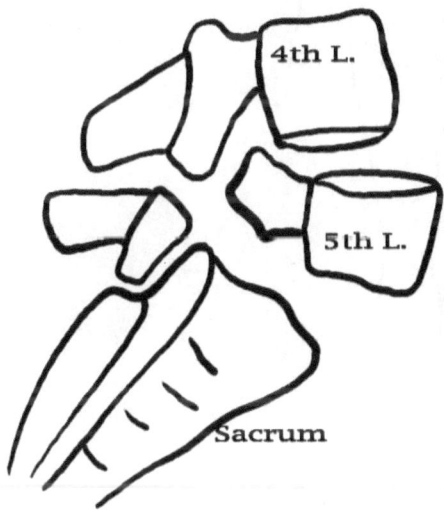

Spondylolisthesis 5th Lumbar Vertebrae

Fig. 10

2. Scoliosis—Congenital or acquired in adolescence. It is an abnormal curvature of the spine, with some rotation of the vertebra (frontal and transversal plane). Early orthopedic aggressive treatment is necessary to avoid further deformity, especially in the female with its cosmetic consequences; again, pain of mechanical origin.

    This condition requires close orthopedic supervision (fig.12).

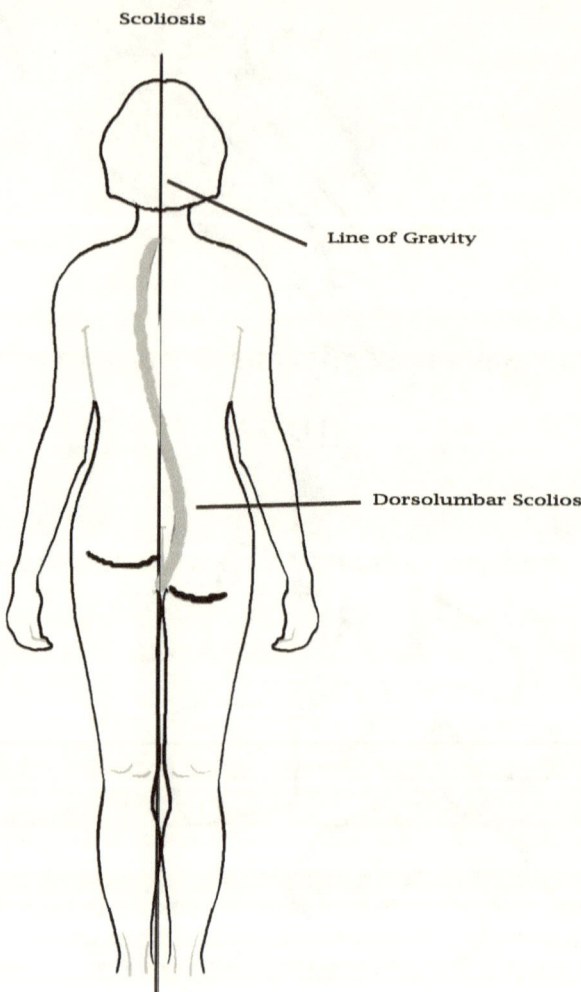

Fig. 12

3. Adolescent osteochondrosis—Scheuermann's disease (condition described by this physician in 1936) is due to a prolapse of the nucleus of a disc into the body of the above or below vertebral body, so-called Schmorl node (1927). Again, this condition needs close orthopedic supervision.

4. Spina bifida occulta—Due to an abnormality of the neural canal caused by a defective closure of the vertebral column. I am only talking of the benign type (not the complete open spine seen at birth with severe neurological deficit). Again this condition needs close medical treatment (fig. 13).

Spina Bifida Occulta

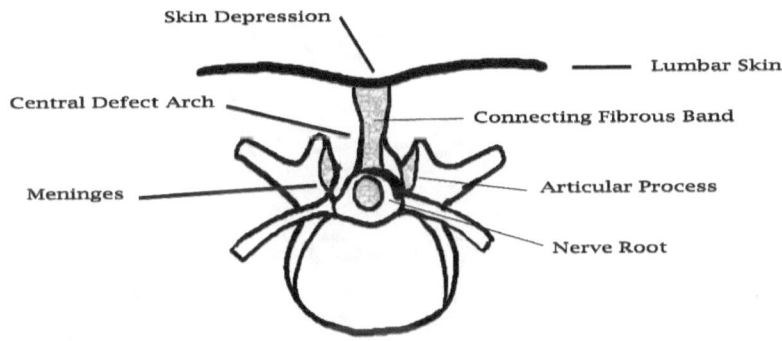

Fig. 13

5. Sacralization of the fifth lumbar vertebra—The vertebra is fused to the sacrum and looks like part of the sacrum. It is a benign developmental condition capable of causing low back pain.

6. Lumbarization of the first sacral segment—The upper part of the sacrum is separated from the rest and looks like a lumbar vertebra, with the formation of a disc space. Again, a developmental condition, which could cause low back pain (fig. 14 and 15).

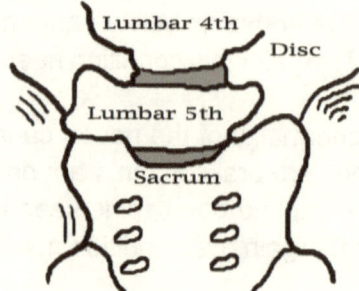

Sacralization of the
Transverse Process L5

Hemisacralization of L5

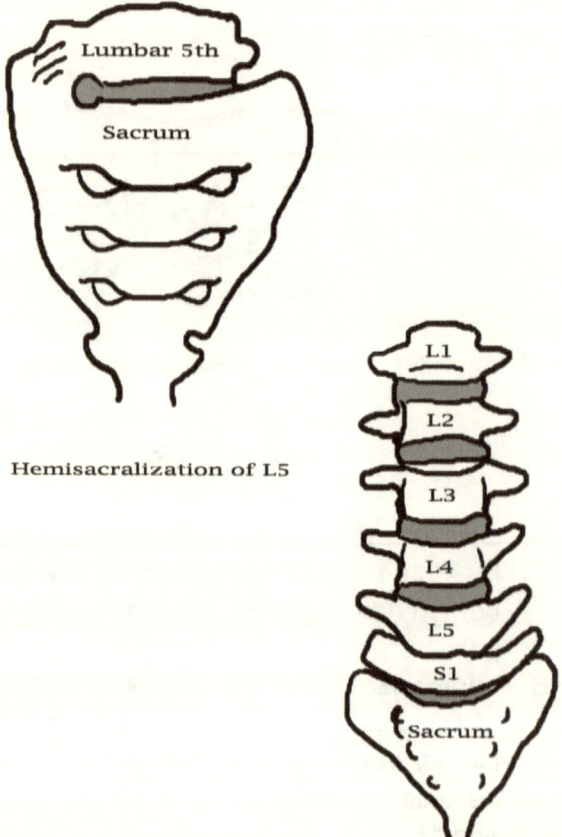

Lumbarization of S1

Fig. 14 & 15

7. Leg discrepancy—Twenty five per cent of individuals do have one leg shorter than the other one

    It is not a cause of backache. Normally, a shortening of less than an inch is compensated by a downward pelvic tilt, making both legs equal. The lumbar spine curves, and this is a so-called functional scoliosis. Prescription of a shoe lift is a mistake since it could produce or increase low back pain. A lift should only be prescribed when leg discrepancy is over an inch (2.5 cm).

8. Infection—Osteomyelitis which is a result of a bacteremia (an infection spread from another region), requires emergency medical care and possible surgical intervention

9. Benign tumors—Eosinophilic granuloma, osteoid osteoma, etc. They all require medical orthopedic care.

10. Malignant tumors—From bone, from nerve tissue, or elsewhere, like Wilm's tumor from the kidney, all requiring surgical or medical care.

11. A child can suffer from lumbago, low back pain, and even radiculitis pain going into the leg, due to mechanical reasons different from the ones mentioned above, and the pain may be associated to bending, pushing, stooping, or lifting.

12. Herniated lumbar disc is rare. The treatment is essentially conservative Non-surgical. The treatment will be the same as the conservative treatment of the low back pain in an adult, which will be described in the following chapters.

Chapter 3

Adult Lower Back Pain

Lumbago is a challenging and frustrating condition. Usually starting after overuse, bending, pushing, lifting, stooping, or minimal rotation like an off-balance movement of the lower back.

The pain could be located in the middle of the lumbosacral region (central), on one side (unilateral), or both sides (bilateral). Sometimes, pain follows a clicking sensation; the nature of the pain could vary from a dull to a sharp intensity.

An examination will show a spasm of the lumbosacral muscles, and the patient adopts a position called "antalgic scoliosis," according to Steindler (The reversibility of low back pain and sciatic symptoms and their relation to the antalgic attitudes, Schweizerische Medizinische Wochchenschrift, 1954, No 35, pag.106). The patient is tilted to one side, the contracted muscles act as a splint to immobilize the back and avoid further damage. Motion of the lumbar spine is restricted and painful (flexion, lateral bending, and rotation). There is localized or diffused tenderness to palpation (deep touching) of the lumbar region; we usually find palpable tender points (the patient experiences excruciating pain in a pinpoint area) (fig. 16) called "trigger points." There is no pain in the lower extremities, no neurological deficit (we'll explain this later), normal reflexes, and no sensory changes.

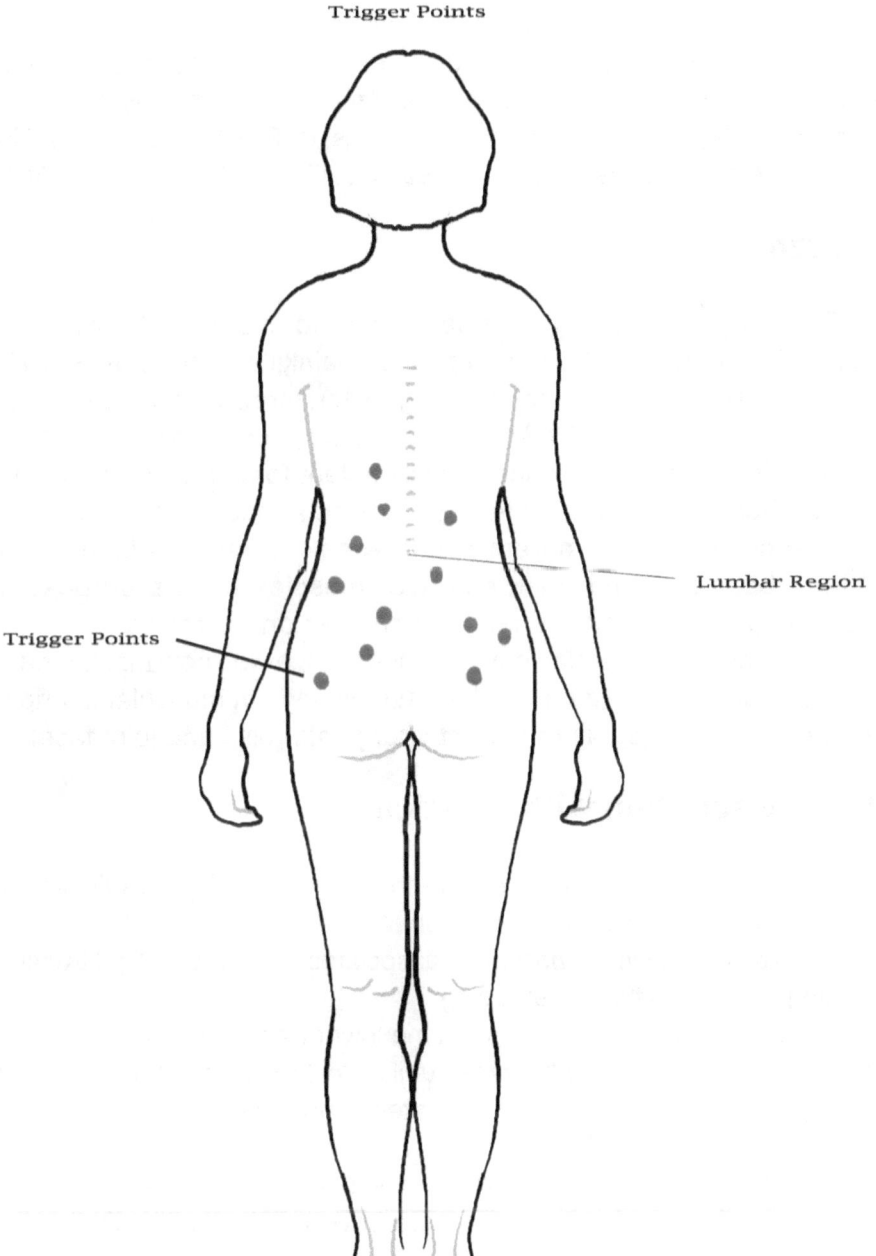

Fig. 16

The diagnosis is low back sprain (which involves the ligaments between the facet joints, vertebra to vertebra, or muscles tendons) or low back strain (involving the lower back muscles).

This is the most common condition. Everyone gets it, sooner or later. I will emphasize that the sprain or strain is localized ONLY in the lower back, no other localization. If the pain extends to the legs, IT IS NOT A BACK SPRAIN. If the pain extends to the abdomen or testicles, IT'S NOT A BACK SPRAIN.

Treatment

This condition usually subsides in four to five days. I advise half a day of bed rest, intake of analgesics (painkillers, such as NSAIDs [nonsteroidal anti-inflammatory drugs]) for three or four days (see chapter about NSAIDs). Avoid bending, pushing, or lifting for two weeks, but remain active. The prognosis is excellent for complete recovery.

For those of sedentary life, I will advise a muscle strengthening/endurance exercise program to increase the strength/endurance of the abdominal and back extensor muscles for the purpose of preventing future back injuries (see chapter on exercises).

The concept of exercise have changed since we know that lumbago and sciatica are in a way "articular" lesions and not muscular in origin, so the exercise's goal is to protect your joints (disc and joint facets).

Acute Back Pain with Sciatica

Back pain extending to one or both lower extremities (radiculitis) is due to an acute herniated lumbar disc.

It can start as a simple backache associated to exertion, slight twisting, bending, pushing, lifting or stooping.

If the pain is localized, at first on the lower back (central, or bilateral) and two or three days later becomes unilateral (one side), then it is almost pathognomonic (indicative) of a herniated lumbar disc. Later on, the pain will move to the leg (radiculitis).

The disc herniation (or rupture) is most commonly seen at the level or between the fourth and fifth lumbar vertebrae or between the fifth lumbar vertebra and the sacrum.

The disc bulges, protrudes, herniates, or ruptures through the posterior vertebral ligament (PVL) (fig. 17) and produces compression over the cauda equina or nerve root, which exit the canal at the foramen level (fig. 18). At the L4/L5 level (fourth lumbar/fifth lumbar) it will compress the Fifth nerve root, and at the L5/S1 (fifth lumbar/first sacral) level, it will compress the S1 nerve root (different symptomatology).

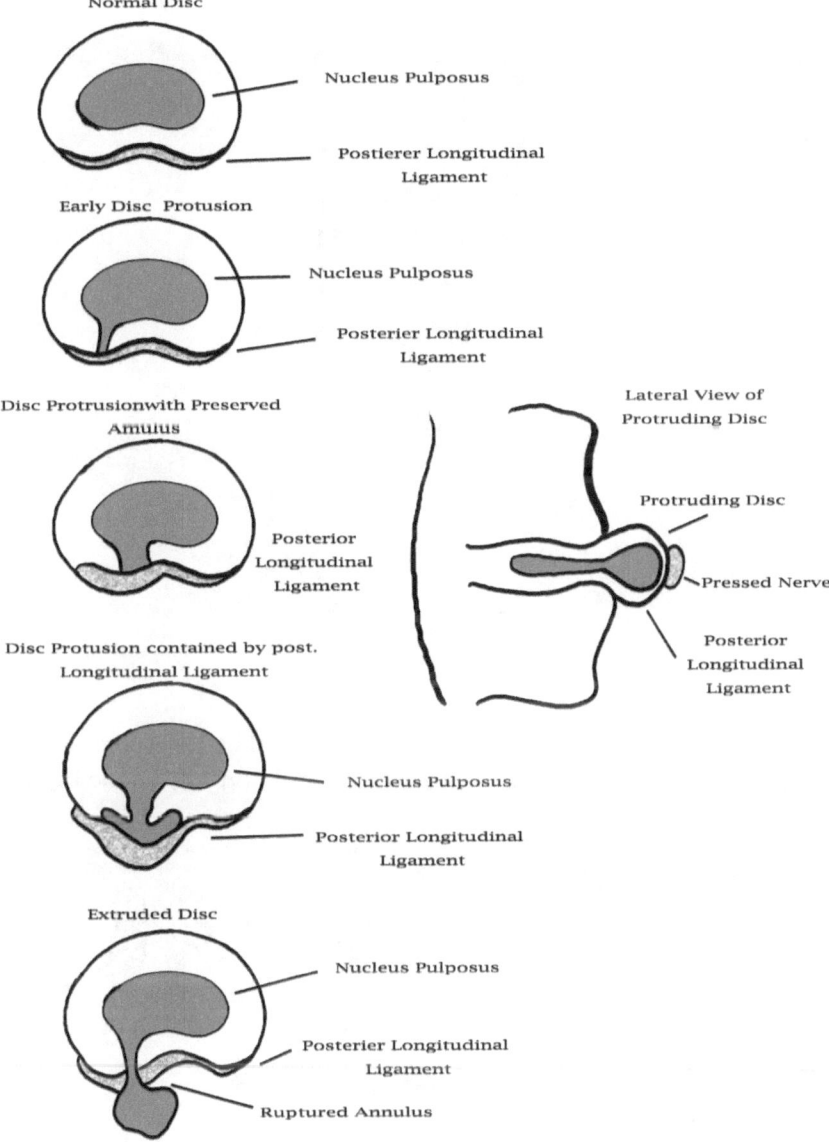

Fig. 17

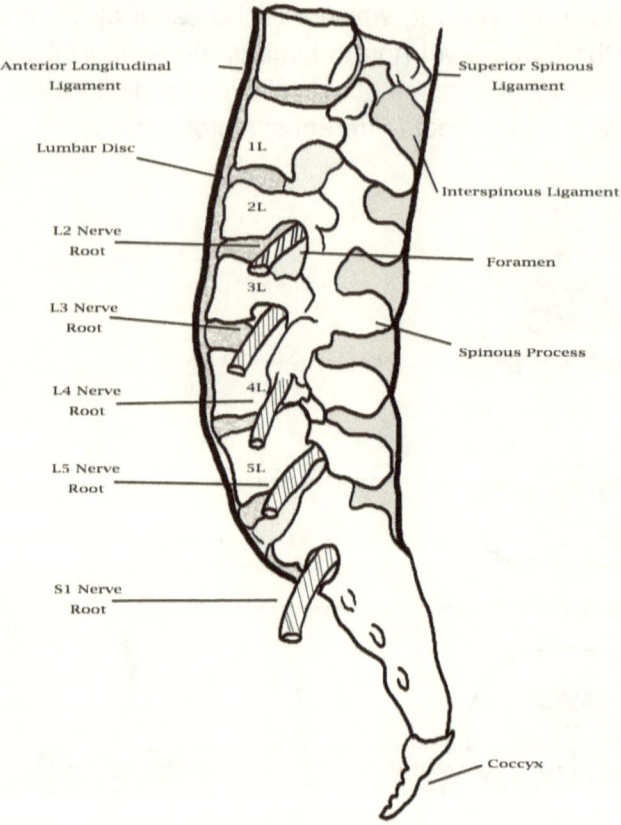

Fig. 18

The protrusion, herniation, or rupture disc could be central or lateral (fig. 19). Fortunately, lateral herniation is the most common. Let's describe them.

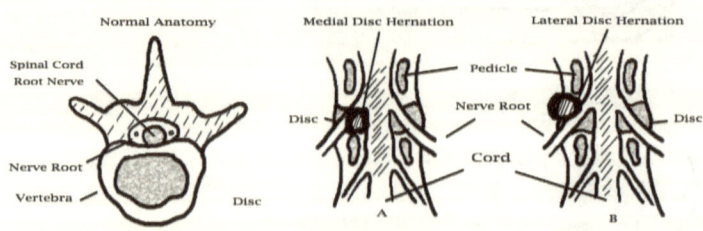

Fig. 19

1. Acute Central Disc Herniation

The disc herniates medial to the nerve root (fig.19), on or about the vertebral midline, compressing the cauda equina (horse tail). The sciatic nerve roots plus the third and fourth sacral roots (bladder) are squeezed on each side.

The symptoms are severe lower back, sacral, and perineal pain (perianal region, buttock), perineal and anus anesthesia, urinary incontinence or paralysis of the bladder, bowel control problems, bilateral radiculitis (pain in both legs, sciatica). Also perineal, hypo (less) or total anesthesia of this area (to touch, pressure, pain, heat, or cold), diminished or abolish reflexes of the legs (knee jerk, ankle jerk). This is a REAL EMERGENCY. Rapid consultation with an orthopedic or neurosurgeon is advised, since IMMEDIATE SURGERY to relieve pressure is necessary.

2. **Acute Lateral Herniated Lumbar Disc** (see fig.19):

It is the most common disc herniation; the disc herniates lateral to the nerve root, almost as it exits the spinal canal (foramen), so symptoms and findings are related to the compression of that nerve root; the right or left fifth nerve root (L4/L5 disc space), and the right or left S1 nerve root (L5/S1 disc space) are the most common disc herniations.

Symptoms are sharp low back pain of any intensity located to one side, both sides, or center of the back region, sometimes like a sharp clicking sensation related to exertion. As mentioned before, a bilateral pain, which after a day or two becomes unilateral, is typical (pathognomonic) of a herniated lumbar disc. One to a few days later, the pain radiates (moves) to a lower extremity. Pain is usually aggravated by coughing or sneezing. Numbness and tingling sensation of the foot and leg may appear (indicating nerve irritation).

Observation of the patient (we call it inspection) will show the patient to be tilted to one side, due to unilateral muscle spasm (antalgic scoliosis); the patient has a painful and restricted motion of lumbar spine, mainly forward flexion. He/she will have a positive straight leg-raising test (fig. 20) where the patient is lying flat on his or her back, the examiner will raise up straight the leg, and the patient will complain at certain angle of excruciated pain on back and leg, indicating nerve root irritation. As an example, a twenty-degree positive angle will indicate more pronounced nerve irritation than at fifty-degree angle, because with this maneuver we stretch the irritated nerve more.

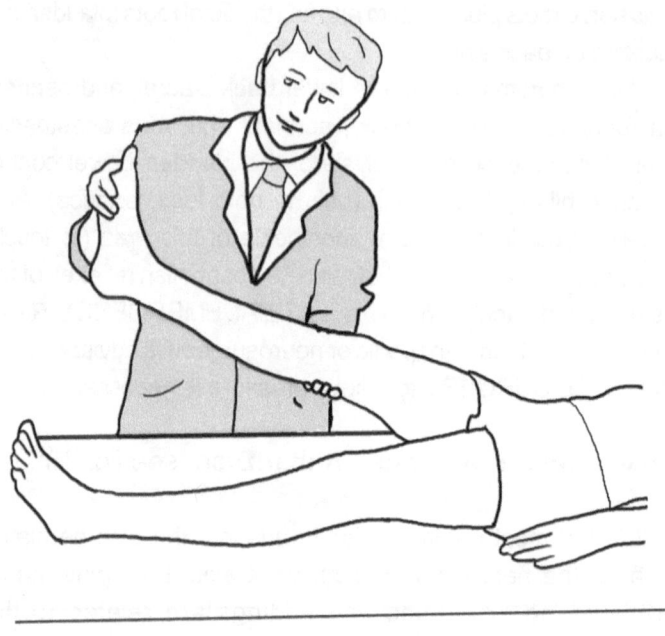

Straight Leg Raising Test

Fig. 20

The patient could have less feeling to touch and prick on the medial aspect of the painful leg (area of the big toe) on the L4/L5 disc or in the outer aspect of the foot (area of the little fifth toe) on the L5/S1 disc (fig. 21). As the condition progresses, the patient could develop muscle weakness, difficulty to stand on tiptoes, or on his or her heels on the affected side (fig. 22).

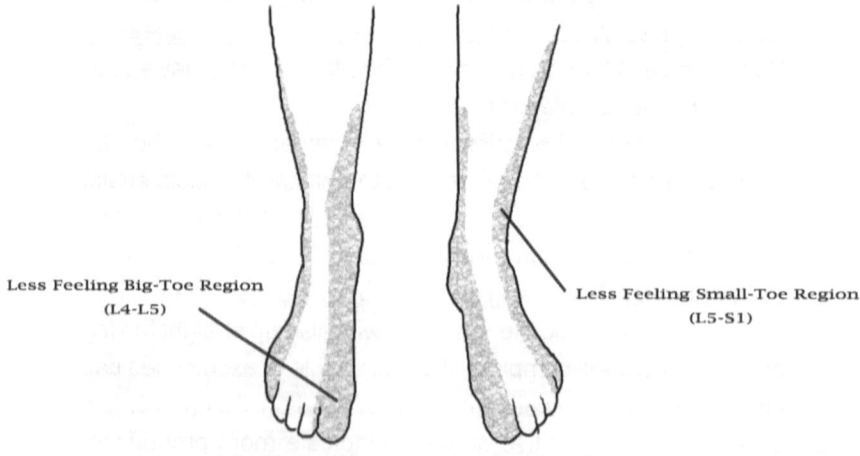

Less Feeling Big-Toe Region (L4-L5)

Less Feeling Small-Toe Region (L5-S1)

Fig. 21

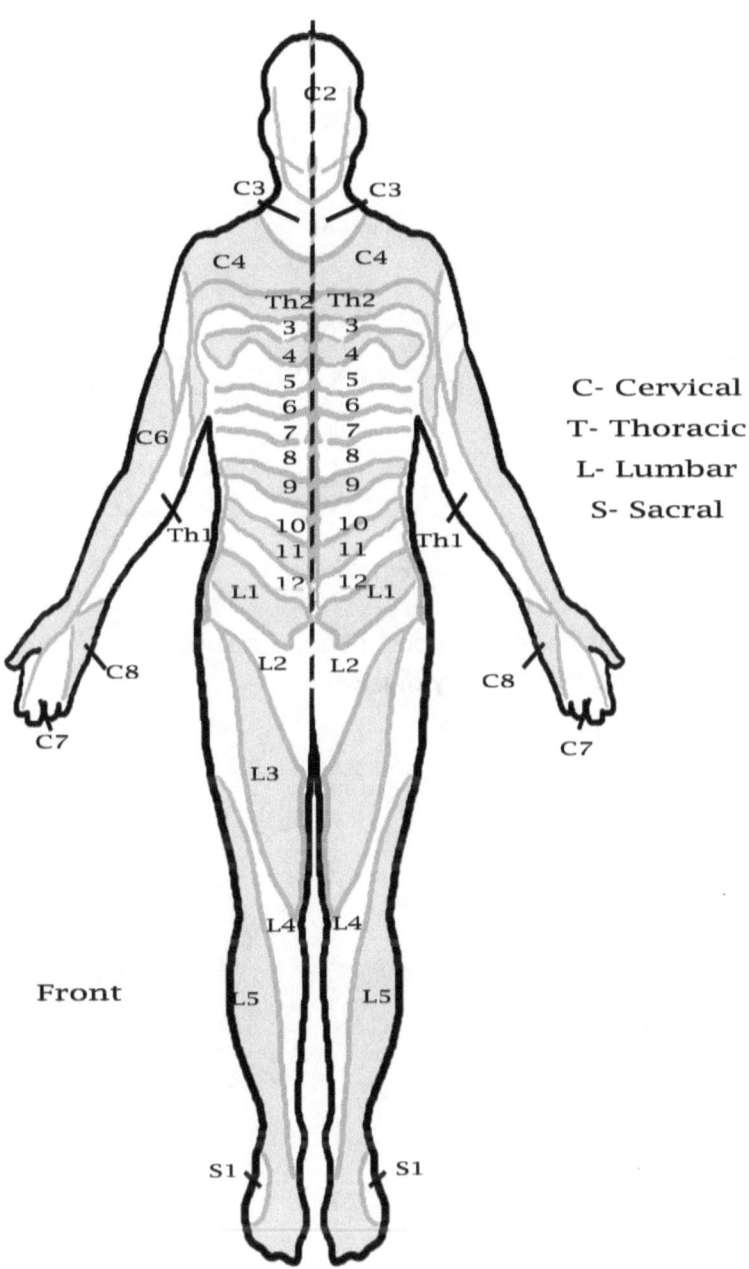

Nerve Root Distributiom

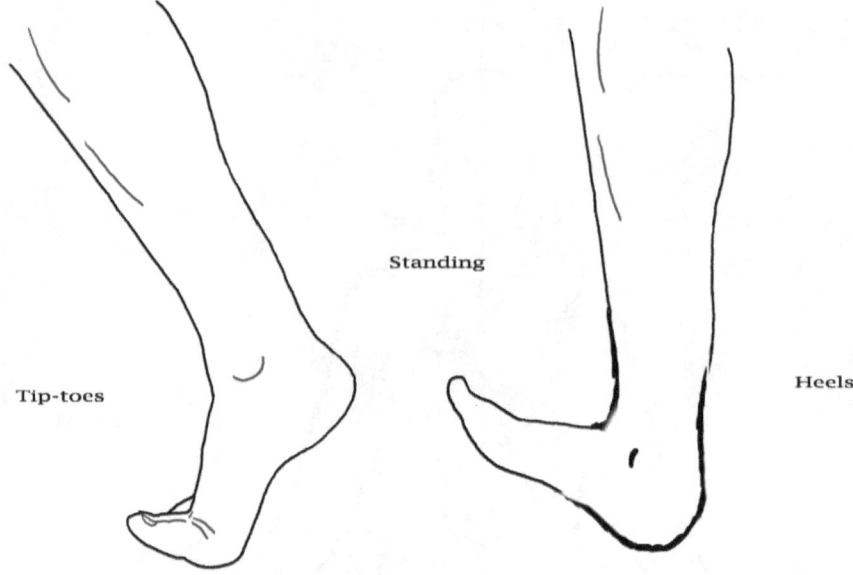

Fig. 22

The knee or ankle reflexes could be diminished or abolished for the fourth or fifth discs respectively (fig. 23).

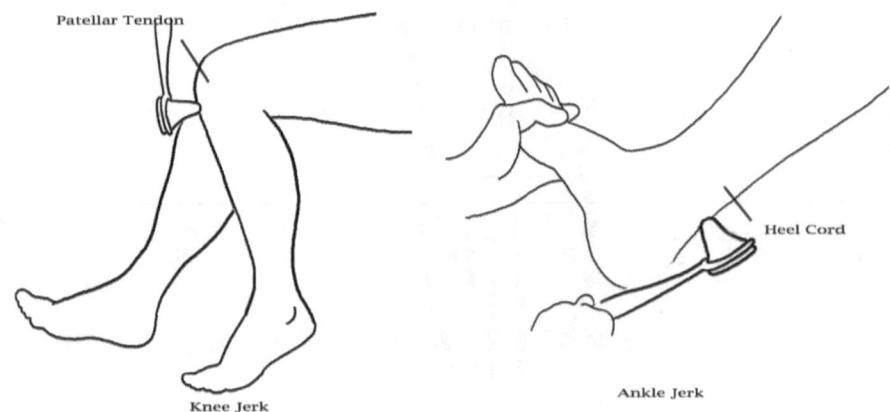

Fig. 23

Studies to Confirm Diagnosis

Plain x-rays of the lumbosacral spine will be negative. Regular x-rays only show bones, a disc is a soft tissue structure. However, plain x-rays are the first step to any further study in order to rule out any other pathology.

Computerized Tomography (CT). These studies will show a herniated or ruptured disc. CT uses radiation. It shows excellent bone, soft tissue, and disc images.

Anthropometrics CT studies have shown the importance of intervertebral disc size in low back pain. The average size of the vertebral disc was significantly smaller in people with low back problems (CMJ, Clinical Sciences, 45(6): 734-739, 2004).

Lumbar myelogram. Intrathecal injection by way of a spinal puncture of a contrast material (into the dural space). It will show notching of the thecal membrane due to a herniated or ruptured disc (distortion of the fluid-filled sheath surrounding the spinal canal). However, this is a painful procedure and is not necessary to diagnose an HLD (herniated lumbar disc) since the MRI came into the picture.

Magnetic resonance image (MRI) is the method of choice, being painless and showing the exact pathology.

Other advantages to a CT are that it's a nonradiation study and provide better images of soft tissues, bone marrow, neural element, and vertebral bone. Of course there are cases where this procedure is contraindicated, especially if the patient has metal or a pacemaker in his/her body, so a CT is the answer in those cases.

CAUTION, CAUTION

"Substantial percentages of individuals who never had low back pain or sciatica but had abnormal myelograms (24%), computerized tomography scans (CT) (36%), or discograms (37%) have been reported. In the present study (JBJS, Vol. 72-A, NO. 3, March 1990, pp 403-408, Abnormal Magnetic-Resonance Scans of the Lumbar Spine in

Asymptomatic Subjects, By Boden, S.D, Davis, D. O. and coll.), about 30% of an asymptomatic population (no signs of low back pain) had a major abnormality on a magnetic resonance image (MRI). The finding that an asymptomatic individual has more than a one-in-four chance of having an abnormal magnetic resonance image (MRI) emphasizes the danger of predicting a decision to operate on the basis of any diagnostic tests in isolation, without clinical information. A diagnosis that is based on magnetic resonance image (MRI), in the absence of objective clinical findings, may not be the cause of the patient's pain, and an attempt at operative correction could be the first step toward disaster.

Well that is so far in terms of diagnosis

How Do We Treat an Acute Herniated Lumbar Disc?

Surgical or Non-Surgical (Conservative)?

My experience is that only about 5% of patients with herniated lumbar disc (HLD) will need surgery (lumbar laminectomy and excision of protruding herniated disc). Against popular knowledge, SURGERY is NOT NECESSARY, except in those cases with marked neurological deficit, like paralysis or "drop foot" where the patient cannot bring the foot up at the level of the ankle joint (dorsiflexion), and the foot drops when walking.

The patient with "drop foot" will compensate by bending high the thigh and knee, when walking. Even this functional impairment could be corrected by a small brace. By the way, it is only probable that the patient with peroneal palsy (drop foot) will recuperate after surgery; by the same token, I have patients that regained complete function just with conservative treatment, using a brace and physical therapy.

Cyriax (Textbook of Orthopaedic Medicine, sixth Edition) said that there are few ways in which spontaneous recovery is secured; one way is by reduction, where the displaced part of the disc may return to its bed spontaneously, easing the pressure over the nerve root. Another way, by erosion, the disc fragment erodes the vertebral bone and accommodates to this new position, with no more root nerve pressure, and the patient recovers fully (fig. 24).

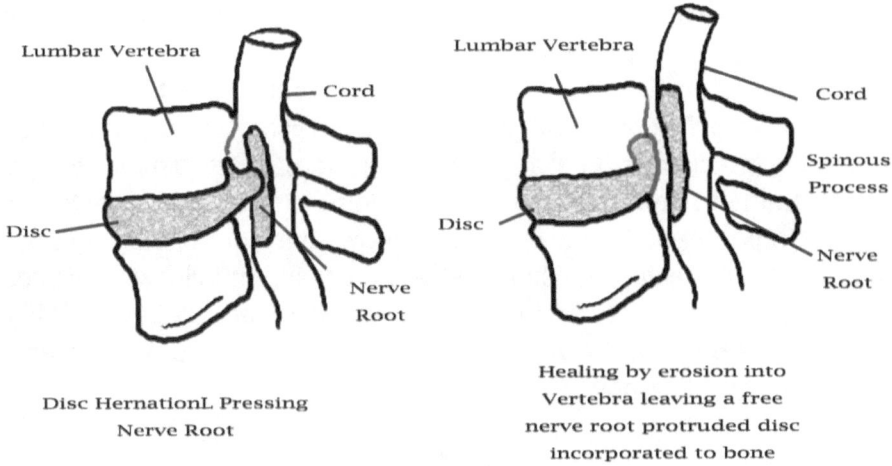

Disc HernationL Pressing
Nerve Root

Healing by erosion into
Vertebra leaving a free
nerve root protruded disc
incorporated to bone

Fig. 24

"We learn from Schmorl and Junghanns as well from many others, that the degenerated disc may heal by fibrous scar, even after some of its mass has penetrated epidurally (protrusion, extrusion, ruptured disc), and that this results in a "functional quiescence," meaning spontaneous shrinking with pain subsiding.

Conservative treatment may cause a ruptured or extruded disc to shrink to 1/5 of its original size" (Schweizerische Medizinische Wochenschrift, # 35, pg.1016, The reversibility of low back and sciatic symptoms and their relation to the antalgic attitudes. A. Steindler).

Conservative Treatment Is the Treatment of Choice

An acute disc herniation is treated as follows:

1. **Bed rest** for a short period of three to five days. "Rest is the commonest treatment prescribed after analgesics (painkillers) but is based on a doubtful rationale, and there is little evidence of any lasting benefit. There is, however, little doubt about the harmful effects especially of prolonged bed rest. Conversely, there is not evidence that activity is harmful; and contrary to common belief, it does not necessarily make the pain worse" (PMID: 2961080,1987

Volvo Award in Clinical Sciencies, Orth. Dept., Western Infirmary, Glasgow, Scotland).

2. **Active motion** and gentle back exercises in the three planes: forward flexion, (always painful and restricted in a herniated lumbar disc); extension (backward flexion); lateral bending to right and left and rotating to right and left are the key for treatment. "Experimental studies clearly show that controlled exercises not only restore function, reduce distress, and illness behavior, and promote return to work, but actually reduce pain" (PMID: 2961080,1987 Volvo Award in Clinical Sciences, Orth. Dept., Western Infirmary, Glasgow, Scotland).

How far should she or he move?

(1) With a slow start, increase range of motion progressively as improving. (2) Range of motion should stop when pain appears. Chapter 10 discusses my isometric/endurance program of exercises; also, I recommend at the beginning to perform the exercises twenty minutes after ingestion of analgesics.

3. **Intake of analgesics** (painkillers)—nonsteroidal anti-inflammatory drugs (NSAIDs)—at proper dose (therapeutic dose) after meals to protect your gastrointestinal tract (GI). Sometimes the patient will require narcotics for two or three days (see special chapter).

4. **Physical Therapy** and gentle manipulations, in my personal experience, is not needed. However, there are special cases where a patient needs to be guided with physical therapy (depressed, unwilling to comply, unable to understand nature of treatment, lazy, and those under workmen's compensation cases where there is some gain by being disabled). I am not against the application of heat or ice. I am not against electrical stimulation, TENS units (transcutaneous electrical nerve stimulation), ultrasound, or acupuncture. I repeat: these are not necessary.

RETURN to WORK as SOON as POSSIBLE three to four weeks for those of sedentary work. Labor workers should return in about six weeks, the first three months should be on light duty. They should perform minimal bending, pushing or lifting, and no stooping.

I advise the wearing of support: a lumbosacral corset, just for work only. After three months, an assessment of heavy work should be performed. I recommend a back school for those engaged in labor work, under a highly reputable physical medicine professional who will determine if there is any partial or total permanent functional impairment due to the residual low back condition.

Future of a Person Who Suffered a Herniated Lumbar Disc

My experience and so of others is that anybody that sustained a herniated or ruptured disc has some unknown "intrinsic" weakness of the lumbosacral spine and a propensity to a recurrence within one to three years. He/she will be more vulnerable to any minimal trauma, which will prolong any period of recovery.

Definitely, they will develop early degenerative osteoarthritis (arthrosis) of the spine, involving discs, facet joints, what I will call "early aged."

My advice is to those patients to change habits of life. If he/she performs heavy work like physical labor type, definitely should retrain for another type of job, even with less remuneration. Otherwise, later on, for obvious reasons, it will be more costly.

For those engaging in sedentary work, they should become more active and get involved in a program of exercises or sports, which do not require sudden involuntary motions like pivoting in basketball or tennis. I advise walking, jogging, and swimming among others.

Surgery vs. Conservative Treatment. Several studies in this country and abroad showed that after one or two years, the surgical or non-surgical patient is clinically the same.

"Lumbar diskectomy is the most common surgical procedure for back and leg symptoms, but the efficacy of the procedure relative to nonoperative care remains controversial" (James N Weinstein and coll. JAMA.2006; 296:2441-2450).

My opinion is that those treated conservatively do much better (including myself).

Surgery brings the potential of several complications like anesthesia (rare, but it happens); infections (rare, but do happen); neurological, like a "drop foot" (paralysis of the peroneal nerve); and the worse (not to enumerate all of them), meningeal scarring of the dura matter, a terrible complication, result of a physiological response of your body, different in each person, a real nightmare of intractable pain, which might require possibly several major surgical interventions.

Summing It Up

Treatment of acute herniated or ruptured disc should be conservative in 98% of cases.

Chapter 4

Chronic Low Back Pain in the Middle Age

I call chronic low back pain when episodes of low back pain come and go over a period of six months or more (with or without radiculitis: sciatica).

In those patients, ligaments and muscles are affected; ligaments have become inelastic due to recurrent sprains (scars from healed microfiber ruptures), and short and long muscles have scars in the insertion points or in the muscle mass due to recurrent strains (partial tears).

The vertebral joints degenerate and become arthritic (irregular instead of smooth); the disc spaces collapses, due to disc degeneration, loss of water, and elasticity; the jelly-like center of the disc often dries out; the strong fibers of the annulus weaken and tear; and there is formation of bone spurs (osteophytes) in the periphery of the vertebral bodies and facet joints (fig. 25).

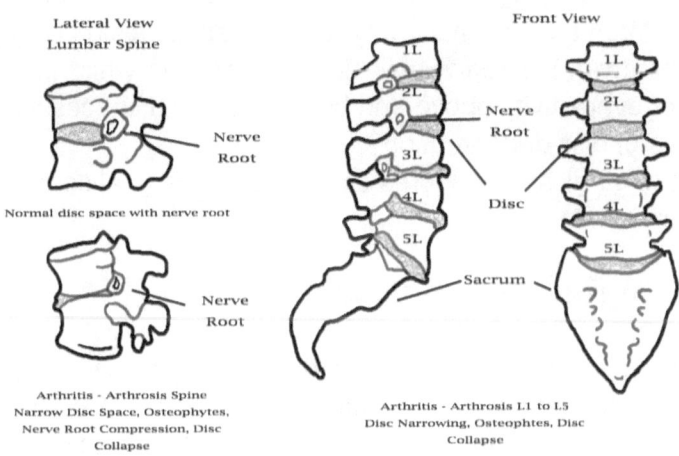

Fig. 25

We are dealing now with a permanent disease. Its symptoms will depend on the degree of degeneration of each structure. Now we have somebody with "a weak back" (as people like to call it).

The patient may show an increase of the normal lumbar lordosis (backward concavity) especially if overweight.

The back pain is present and could be associated to exertion. There is restricted and painful motion of the lumbosacral spine, tenderness over muscles and ligaments, trigger-point areas, decreased or abolished reflexes, positive or negative "stretching test for the sciatic nerve" (straight leg raising test) (fig. 20). The low back pain could be radiated or not to the right or left lower extremities, with or without numbness and tingling sensation in the legs.

X-ray examinations (I advise complete x-rays studies: anteroposterior, lateral, and right and left oblique, otherwise you could miss some pathology) will show degenerative changes of the vertebral joints, marked narrowing of disc spaces, and bony spurs (fig. 25).

MRI will be positive to show degenerative osteoarthritis and "hard disc" protrusions encroaching the cord.

EMG (electromyography) study of the muscles' contractions, which assesses muscle function, most of the time, shows the presence of radiculitis.

We are now dealing with a patient who showed marked pathology (abnormalities).

What do we do? An inexperienced surgeon will advise surgery.

What a mistake! Is he able to correct by way of surgery all these multiple conditions, by removing a hard disc with a laminectomy, or preventing intervertebral motion by way of a spinal fusion (using a bone graft and hardware), or replacing it by disc prosthesis, which in a few years because of overactivity above and below the fused spaces will create a worse case of disc degeneration?

All these surgical procedures can create meningeal scarring—a real medical nightmare.

Treatment Recommended

Say no to surgery except those cases of extreme neurological deficit like an acute paralysis of an extremity.

You should understand that you suffer from a chronic low back pain, a "weak back," and you have to learn to live with it.

This is not the end of the world. You will live a normal life; you will be able to engage in certain sports like walking, jogging, swimming, bicycling, or golfing.

Let's go to real treatment:

1. Keep your weight down by eating properly (everything but with moderation).
2. Wear a lumbosacral support (corset) for protection during activities that require mild amount of bending, pushing, or lifting. Avoid heavy lifting or stooping.
3. During any flare-up take NSAIDs, after each meal as already mentioned, for no more than four to five days.
4. Get involved in a strengthening/endurance program of exercises to increase the strength/endurance of abdominal and back extensor muscles, which will protect your facets and disc joints, which are "the key" of the lumbosacral region.
5. Your examination may show trigger points, painful tender pinpoint areas. (fig. 16). Local infiltrations (injection) of these areas with local anesthetic like 1% xylocaine or 0.5 % mercaine are advised. These infiltrations are harmless (check if you are not allergic) and can be repeated several times a year. Unfortunately, there are each time less physicians who will take the time to perform infiltrations of trigger points. We do not know the pathophysiology (how these injections work); there are many theories (the important fact is that works). At this time, I would like to mention the professor who advocated them over fifty years ago and wrote so much about this subject, Arthur Steindler, MD. He was professor of orthopaedic surgery at the University of Iowa. I had the privilege of undergoing part of my training with him.
6. There are patients where the radicular pain does not improve or subside in spite of the above indicated measures. In these patients, I recommend to undergo three "epidural blocks," in a period of three months (a mix of local anesthetic and steroid, injected at the exit of the nerve's roots). **Advise:** Be sure it is done by a certified anesthesiologist, who is familiar with this type of procedure.
7. Physical therapy and its multiple modalities (heat, ice, gentle massage, electrical stimulation, TENS unit, ultrasound, hydrotherapy, gentle manipulation, etc.). Physical therapy is useful for a short period of time, and it also helps to teach the patient to

carry a program of exercises at home. Again, this should be carried
out by a certified department of physical medicine; I do not feel a
family doctor's office could offer this service.

8. Acupuncture. I read and took courses in acupuncture in this country
   in the former Hahnemann University and in Tokyo, Japan, with
   the purpose of just only to understand its principles and be able
   to prescribe it to my patients. My experience taught me that while
   some patients will have some relief and marked improvement,
   others would not. **My Advise:** Getting acupuncture WILL NOT
   HARM You. So why don't you try it?

Chapter 5

Back Pain in the Elderly

Back pain at this age is a common finding, even without previous history of back pain in adulthood.

The normal process of aging weakens our ligaments and muscles by degenerative changes, and they lose strength. Bones, due to low hormones production, do lose mass (osteoporosis), so they become weaker; the intervertebral discs, due to loss of water content and loss of elastic fibers, collapse. The shock absorber properties of the discs are lost. In the x-rays, due to the discs' collapse you see one vertebra closer to the above and below segment (fig. 26), a hard disc may protrude into the spinal canal; the vertebral bodies do respond with the formation of spurs (osteophytes). The vertebral joints lose its smooth surface (hyaline cartilage) interfering with motion. A small ligament, which extends from one laminae to another laminae (flavum ligament) (fig. 26) will retract as the vertebra become closer and could protrude into the spinal canal.

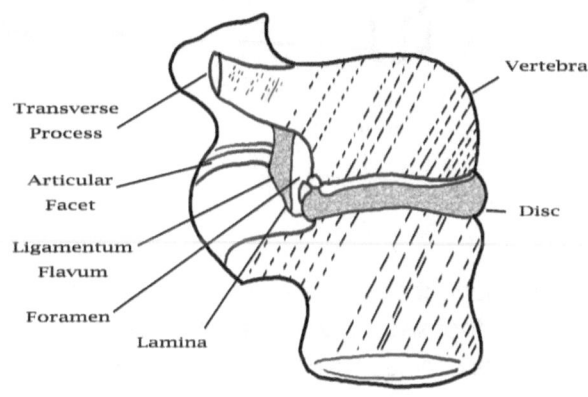

Fig. 26

The circumference of the spinal canal becomes smaller with possible impingement of the cauda equina or nerve roots.

It is very common at this age group to see a narrowing of the circumference of the spinal canal, a condition called spinal stenosis, with signs and symptoms due to compression of the cord or nerve roots.

Spinal stenosis (fig. 27), as I just said, is a common condition of the elderly; the patient suffers of low back pain that extends to the lower extremities, may also have sensations like numbness, pins and needles, tingling; all these symptoms occurring only when walking and being relieved by sitting.

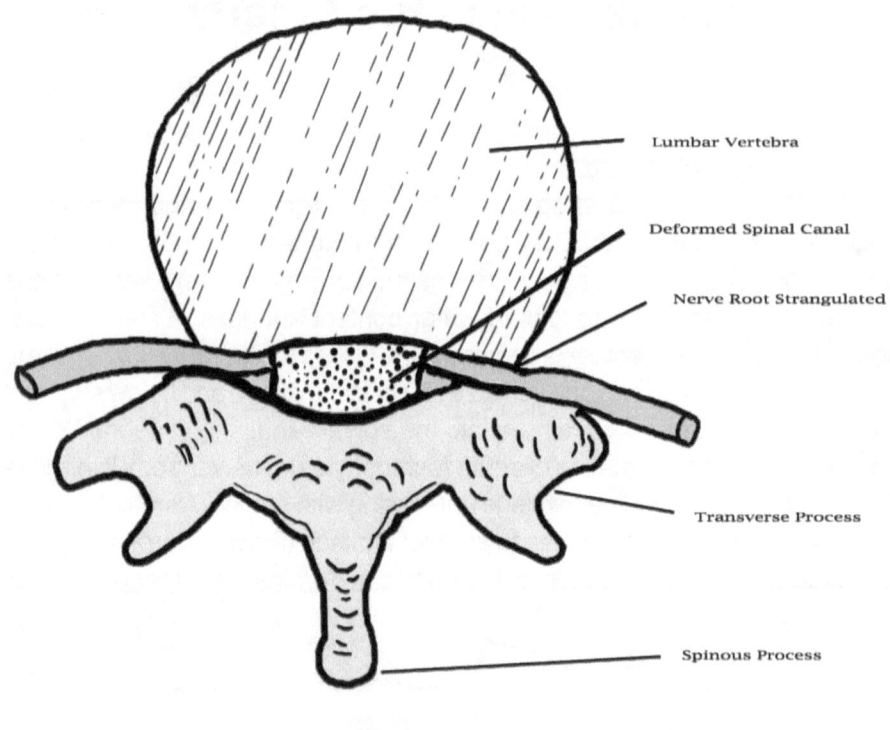

Lumbar Vertebra

Deformed Spinal Canal

Nerve Root Strangulated

Transverse Process

Spinous Process

Spinal Stenosis

Fig. 27

We say that the patient shows "pseudoclaudication," the kind of pain which resembles with that seen in diseases of the leg's arteries (peripheral vascular disease). This condition is not due to impaired vascular circulation of the legs; patients do have adequate arterial circulation, and ultrasound studies of the leg's arteries are normal, showing no obstruction of the arteries.

There is a theory that this condition could occur as a consequence of a sudden and temporary ischemia (insufficient blood supply) to the nerve roots.

Summing up an easy diagnosis: low back pain extending to the legs when walking, and with rapid relief by sitting.

Pain is also relieved by bending forward, and aggravated by bending backward (flexion and extension of the lumbosacral spine) in a standing position, contrary to the findings of a herniated lumbar disc. So forward flexion (bending forward), is a comfortable position for these patients, which in time becomes a permanent type of posture. Now you know one of the reasons why some older people walk bended.

The treatment is CONSERVATIVE. I advise to follow the same treatment as that advised in chronic low back pain in adulthood.

I would like to add that paradoxically the use of a treadmill or bicycling is painless—excellent exercise for spinal stenosis—the reason in these exercises the patient adopt a flexed position, which relieves nerve root compression.

Rarely, the pain is so intense, that the patient can hardly walk. I do feel that in these cases surgery is indicated, what we call a "decompressive laminectomy"(fig. 42). The purpose of surgery is to relieve pain and not to treat a paralysis or other neurological deficit.

Most of the time the stenosis extends to more than one vertebral space, two or three segments, for example from L3 (third lumbar) to S1 (first sacral segment).

Fortunately, an MRI (magnetic resonance image) or a CT scan (computerized tomography) will show exactly the length of the narrow spinal canal to decompress. Spinal fusion, with bone graft plus hardware, as a rule, is not the recommended surgical procedure. At this age, the patient will not engage in a heavy or laborious work, and so we will cut the time of surgery, and avoid postsurgical complications of a spinal fusion.

There is a new surgical treatment, still under trial by the FDA (US Food and Drug Administration); it mainly consists of a distracting device, between two vertebrae, that mechanically gives "more room" to the "pinched" nerve root, relieving the spinal stenosis. One of these devices is the X-Stop made of titanium. It is a small surgical procedure, which can be done under local anesthesia. The surgical indication will of course depend of how many vertebrae are involved and how much stenosis or nerve root compression is present.

Pain in the elderly should be carefully evaluated. If pain is related to motion and activity, it points toward spinal stenosis. Low back pain, which is not relieved by rest or wakes up the patient, should require a thorough medical workup, mainly to rule out the spreading of "a silent tumor" (like prostate in men, breast in women, multiple myeloma, etc.) or a condition like Paget's disease.

Chapter 6

Sacroiliac Sprain

I would like to say a few words about this condition. Contrary to popular and old knowledge, a lesion of the sacroiliac joints and ligaments is rare.

The upper body of the sacrum articulates (a joint) with the right and left ilium bone (os ilei) forming the right and left sarcroiliac joints (the back portion of the pelvis) (fig. 28). It is a kidney shaped joint, and as a joint is subject to any pathology as any other joint. This articulation has motion, like rotation, which may decrease with age and increase due to hormonal effect in the pregnant woman, to prepare the widening of the pelvic ring for delivery. The sacroiliac ligaments protect these joints. Symptoms of a sacroiliac sprain are pain over the upper (right or left) inner part of the buttocks, associated to local tenderness to palpation of the sacroiliac ligaments.

Pelvis
Sacrum, Ischion & Pubis

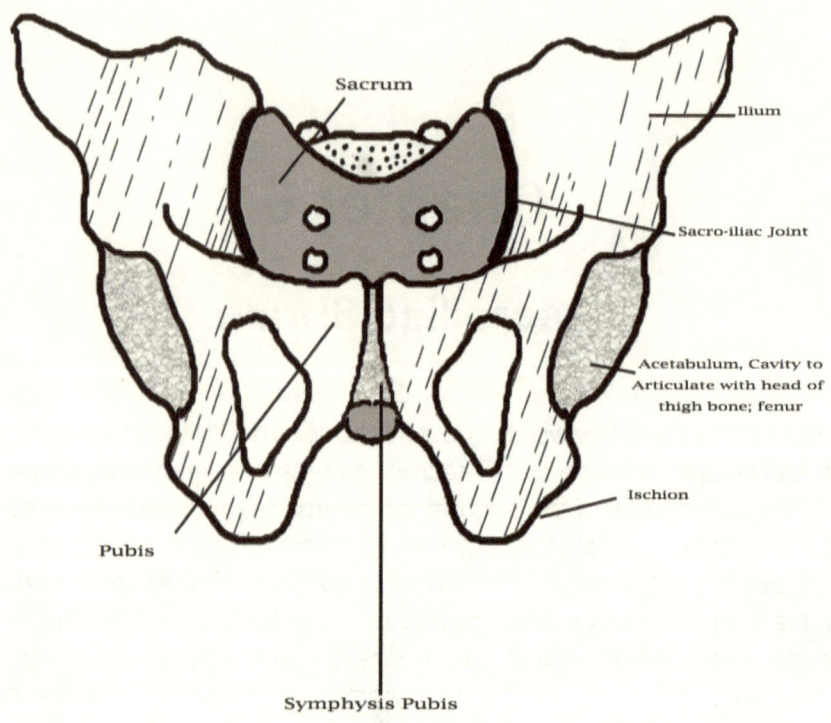

Fig. 28

Subsiding of symptoms, after local anesthetic injection of the tender area, constitutes a diagnostic test for sacroiliac sprain.

The treatment is conservative: intake of analgesics, avoid bending or lifting for few days, and some time local anesthetic infiltration of trigger points.

I would like to point out that rarely chronic sacroiliac sprain could be an early symptom of ankylosing spondylitis, a serious rheumatic condition, since x-rays of these joints could be normal for many years. A rheumatologist should treat it.

Chapter 7

Coccygodynia or Pain on the Tailbone

I just rapidly mention this condition as is closely related to low back pain.

Coccygodynia is a painful coccyx bone (fig. 43). Pain is mainly present when sitting, as vertical compression is applied; by palpation; and sometimes by defecation. Pain tends to be relieved by standing or lying down.

The cause of pain in the tailbone is most of the time local, like when falling in your buttock, or after delivery in women. It is possible to observe radiologically a fracture or a subluxation of the coccyx bone, but the "most known cause is unknown." In medicine whatever is of unknown origin we call it "idiopathic," in this case, it is idiopathic coccygodynia.

The treatment is always *conservative*, with intake of analgesics or NSAIDs for few days, proper cushioning by sitting in a doughnut-type pillow, and avoiding weight bearing on the coccygeal region, especially when driving or sitting for long periods of time. Injection (infiltration), with a mix solution of local anesthetic and a colloidal steroid, is indicated.

Coccygodynia is more frequently seen in women, sometimes accompanied by aversion to coitus, in these cases a psychogenic condition should be ruled out by a certified psychiatrist.

Surgical excision of the coccyx bone is an extremely rare indication, sometimes done when excruciating pain is present at defecation (previous psychiatrist consultation). In my personal experience, surgery is indicated no more than in 0.5 % of cases.

Summing up, coccygodynia, pain on the tailbone, is a benign condition. I mentioned it because in rare cases could it be associated (as a referred pain) from a low back disc condition.

Chapter 8

Considering Any Back Surgery

To the rare patient who needs surgery, this is my advice:

I would like to confess that when I started private practice, after passing my boards (American Board of Orthopaedic Surgery), I used to be hurt when a patient would request a second opinion, after I advised surgery. As I got more "mature," I was glad and happy when a patient did ask for a second opinion. As a matter of fact, I would advise the patient to get a second opinion in all my major surgical cases.

I feel a second opinion is always necessary when contemplating surgery. As in every aspect of life, there is not only one answer for the same problem unless this is an emergency, like in a trauma case.

My second advice is that a board certified physician should perform this consultation (certified by the American Board of Orthopaedic Surgery, American Board of Neurosurgery, or American Board of Neurology). If possible, I do prefer that the consultant belong to the same specialty as the referring surgeon.

The third and last advice is that you should look for a consultant. Try not to get a second opinion by the physician pointed by your surgeon (because as a human, sometimes it is difficult not to agree with a friend). I would prefer if the consultant does not work in the same hospital as your surgeon.

Chapter 9

Conservative Treatments
for Low Back Pain

Physical Exercises

We used to think that exercises that increase the strength of the lower lumbar muscles, flexors, extensors, and rotators will cure or improve low back pain. How muscle strength could cure a degenerative process of the discs or facet joints?

Today, the goal should be to build endurance and muscle strength, which will protect and prevent the facets and disc joints from getting hurt.

I believe that isometric endurance, not muscle strength play a great role in preventing low back pain. I mean isometric endurance, which means the function of a muscle to maintain moderate level of force for prolonged periods of time without showing fatigue. Weight lifters do have strong back muscles, and they get low back pain.

We know now that there is no data or evidence to demonstrate that exercise alone will reduce or cure low back pain. It is my opinion as that of many others that exercises are important as a posture correction; postural dysfunction has been advocated as a cause of chronic back pain. Exercises (endurance/strength type) will increase the resistance and power of the flexor (forward bending) and extensor (backward motion) muscles of the lumbar spine, structures, which in turn will protect the lumbosacral spine, mainly the facets and disc joints, making them less vulnerable to any mechanical stress. Other secondary benefits are to improve attitude, relieve depression, reduce stress, and facilitate sleep.

Before describing my own exercise program, I will mention few others, from an historical point of view.

In 1937, Williams published his flexion exercises (forward bending) to avoid compression of the nerve root at the foramen level (tunnel, place of exit of the nerve root; 1-2 Williams P C Lessons of the lumbosacral pain part 1 &2 JBJS 1937,19:393; 19,690).

Mc Neill. He found that in people with chronic low back pain, the extensor (bending backward) muscles were weaker and of less strength (McNeill T, Warwick D, Anderson G, 1980; 6:529).

Mc Kenzie has proposed that physical exercises shift nuclear material (disc, nucleus) away from the posterior lumbar ligament (fig. 29). This is accomplished by extension exercises (backward bending). This program uses the patient response to repeated lumbar motion (flexion, extension, lateral bending, and rotation) to assess which one reduces the patient's many symptoms. These movements are now combined into an individualized exercise program; the patient "centralizes" (focalizes) the pain and ultimately eliminates his or her symptoms. The motion relieves compression by reducing pressure on the nerve (The Mc Kenzie Approach, a Physician Course, Oct. 12-13, 1990, sponsored by State U. of N. York and the Mc Kenzie Institute).

Disc Motion

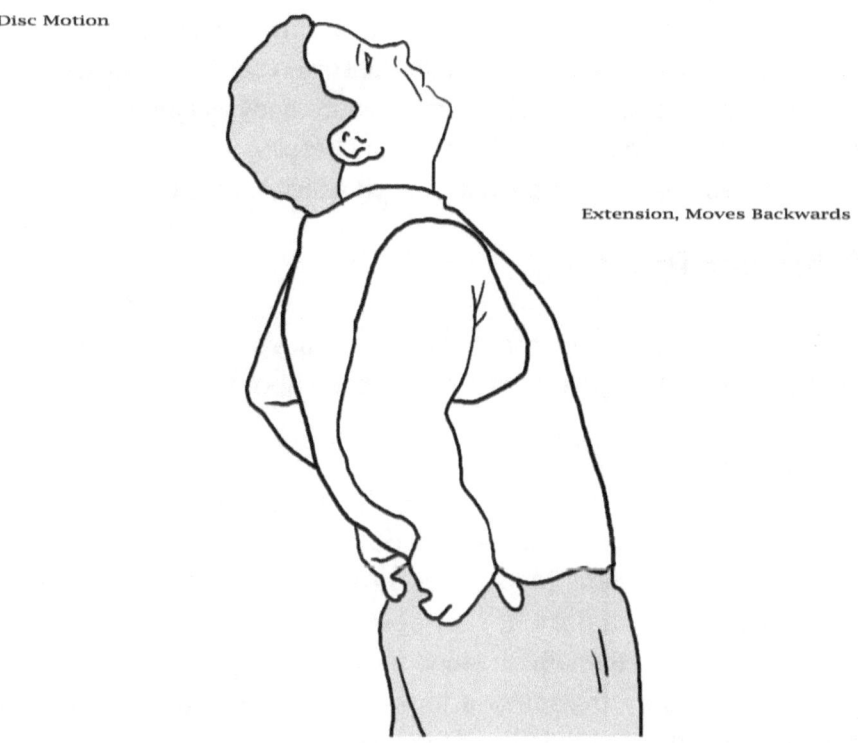

Extension, Moves Backwards

Vertebra

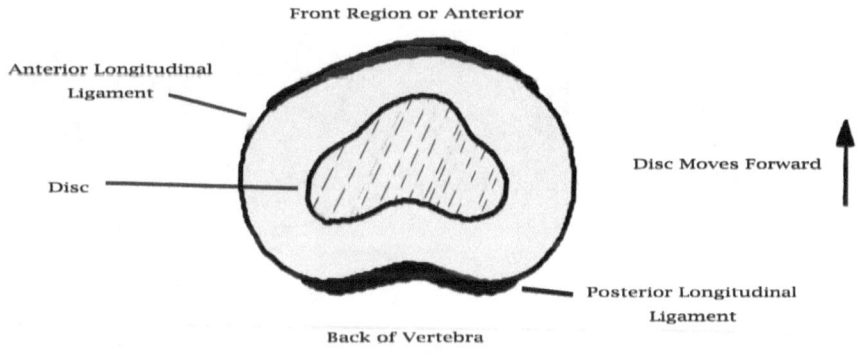

Front Region or Anterior

Anterior Longitudinal
Ligament

Disc

Disc Moves Forward

Posterior Longitudinal
Ligament

Back of Vertebra
or Posterior

Fig. 29

Pelvic Traction

We used to hospitalize a patient and place him in bed with pelvic traction. We used to prescribe a pelvic girdle with eight or ten pounds hanging on each side, but you need at least 25% of the patient's body weight to accomplish any lumbar distraction. So it only helped by keeping the patient in bed. No way you could now admit a patient for such a trivial procedure.

Motorized Traction

Patient on a table and the machine produces pelvic traction. Same comments as with regular traction mentioned above.

90/90 Traction

Advocated by Cotrell (Lancourt J E: traction technique for low back pain (J. Musculoskeletal Med 1986; 3(4): 44-50). The patient while in bed in supine position (face up) is placed with a pelvic sling under his or her buttocks flexing the lumbar spine as much as possible. This position supports the theory that putting tension on the posterior longitudinal ligament (fig. 30) will push forward the disk material. I have no experience with this method and again it could not be performed today as inpatient.

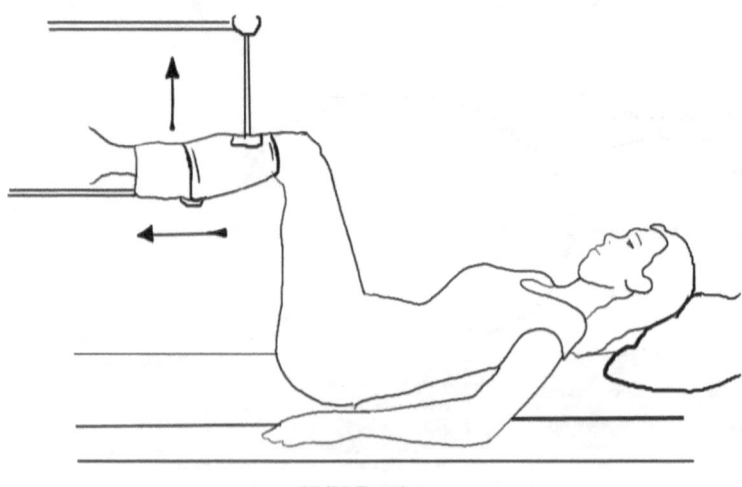

90/90 Traction

Fig. 30

Axial Traction: Sister Kenny introduced the gravity lumbar reduction in 1976. The patient is treated in standing position (fig. 31), placed on an electric-operated tilt bed, fit with a lightweight frame and a specially designed vest that enables the rib cage to serve as a point of fixation. Under supervision, the patient learns how to progressively increase the angle of traction. This regimen is initiated as a hospital inpatient and continued at home (Charles V. Burton, MD, The Journal of MusculoSkeletal Medicine 1986, Pg 12 to 21).

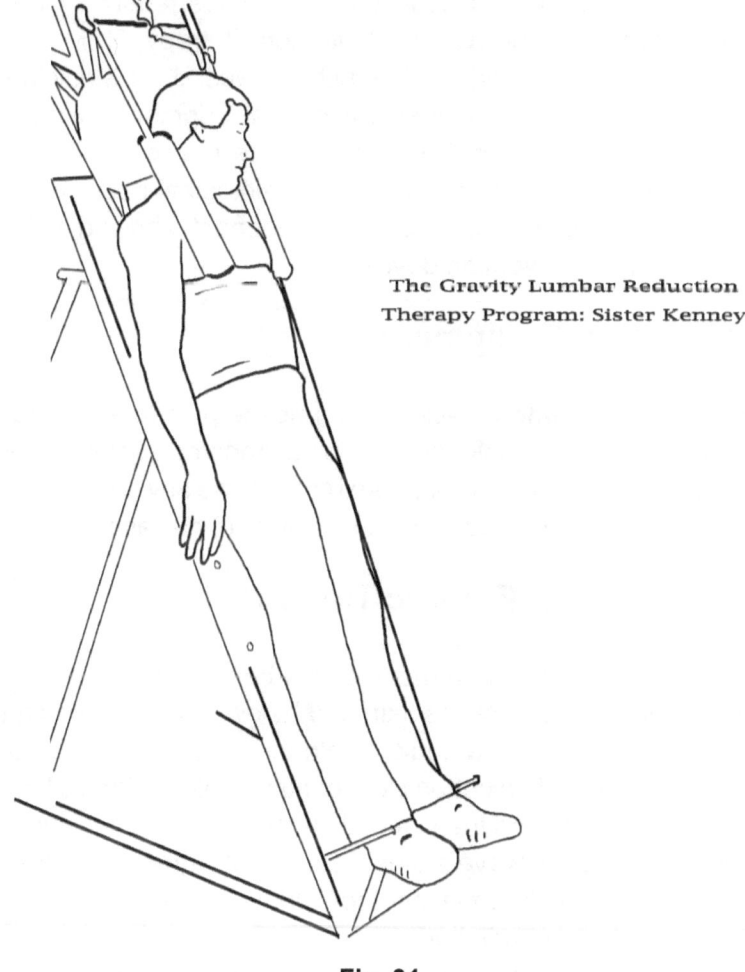

The Gravity Lumbar Reduction
Therapy Program: Sister Kenney

Fig. 31

Today, it would be impossible to admit somebody to a hospital for such a treatment.

Gravity Inversion Therapy

Robert Martin, MD, made gravity inversion therapy popular around 1960. Theoretically, hanging the patient by its ankles and using his or her body weight plus gravity will produce distraction between one vertebra and the other vertebra, causing a decompression, increasing the space between the vertebrae, bringing relief to low back pain. Some of these devices will add oscillation starting in the upright position and going to the 180-degree head down position. Severe complications have been reported, especially if suffering from a heart condition, hypertension, glaucoma, or any other eye condition (Gravity Inversion Therapy; R. M. Klatz, R. M. Goldman, R. S. Tarr, and B. G. Pinchuk, West J. of Medicine.1983 October, 139(4): 538-540). Besides, my clinical judgment will not advise this treatment since there is the need of close medical supervision in case of any emergency with such an unphysiological position. I will be somewhat suspicious to the claims of this treatment, showed in the web, trying to sell a gravity inversion device.

Power Traction Equipment

There is a new method, designed to release pressure on structures that may cause low back pain, called "spinal decompression system."

I have no experience with it; therefore I cannot give any opinion about this treatment. The FDA (Food and Drug Administration) has approved its use.

Heat and Cold, an Empiric Treatment

Heat is another kind of treatment for low back pain.

Regular heat only affects the skin and below fasciae (flat thin tissue covering the muscle), so how could it help the deep structures? Usually it's applied as a hot pack, a cotton cloth container filled with a silicate gel, which is boiled in water and then placed on the lumbar region. Deep heat like diathermia and short wave are applications of high-frequency electric currents. Microwave diathermia, another variation, is a more comfortable form of electromagnetic radiation.

Ultrasound uses high frequency sound waves to penetrate deep; together with infrared light, it will increase blood supply (hyperemia) and even produce swelling; hard to believe, it helps low back pain. Heat gives a nice sensation that is all.

TENS (Transcutaneous Electrical Nerve Stimulation).

Low back pain is alleviated by using a TENS unit attached to the lower lumbosacral region; a battery pack supplies low current and low frequency oscillations, and you feel a gently tingling sensation. Each session, depending on the severity of the pain could last from twenty minutes to few hours.

As a rule, you are taught how to use the unit and to decide for yourself when to apply a treatment. This treatment is contraindicated in patients with severe heart disease, or with a pacemaker, since they could develop a cardiac arrhythmia.

Ice

In my opinion ice is a good analgesic and perhaps a good local muscle relaxant, applied as an ice bag or cold pack. It's called cryotherapy (hard to advise in winter). Similar action can be obtained with the spray of ethyl chloride.

Ice produces vasoconstriction (makes the opening of the arteries to become smaller), excellent as anti-inflammatory for acute trauma.

Massage

Superficial or Deep

1. Superficial, gentle massage is used mainly to relieve swelling or congestion by regular upward stroking. Not for low back pain.
2. Deep Friction to reach deep muscles and deep painful structures, by moving and kneading. It frees adhesions and fibrosis and reduces stress. It is helpful in low back pain.

Contraindications to massage are the following: fever, osteoporosis, or when taking blood-thinning drugs like warfarin (Coumadin).

Manipulation

While many schools have challenged the efficacy of manipulation, it's still one of the most common treatments toward alleviation of low back pain.

We have five different schools of manipulation, as follows: osteopathy, chiropractic, bone setting, oscillation, and orthopaedic medicine (according to James Cyriax).

1. Osteopathy. The object of the manipulation is to restore full range of movement to the spinal joint, based on the idea that all diseases result from vertebral displacements (lack of spinal mobility).
2. Chiropractic means to shift the displaced vertebra back. Chiropractic to place manipulations (adjustments as they call it) are in "fashion" for the treatment of chronic back pain. Perhaps chiropractors spend more time listening to patients. For chronic back pain, manipulations for two or three weeks could alleviate symptoms. However, previously, you should have complete X-ray studies of the lumbosacral spine, a "must" to rule out a tumor, fracture, osteoporosis, and severe osteoarthritis with spinal stenosis. Manipulation in these cases could be a disaster. In manipulations extended over a three-week period, I have seen seems to create like an "addiction" with psychological implications and an "empty pocket."
3. Bone setting—Meaning "click the bones," an inherited profession. You feel or hear a click due to a cartilaginous fragment shift or a snap as an adhesion ruptures, as audible evidence that "bone has been put back." I have no experience on this family related school.
4. Orthopedic medicine advocated by Cyriax, "to get loose fragments of disc back into place." This theory hypothesizes that disc lesions are the primary cause of degenerative changes and pain of the spine. They consist of several maneuvers that I will not describe and which require a specialist in orthopedic medicine or physical medicine. These manipulations are very popular in England. Unfortunately, few physicians in USA put the time to perform this well-probed treatment for low back pain.
5. Oscillation—A rhythmic percussion on a vertebra, pressure and release maneuvers to the affected area; both thumbs are on the tip of spinous process of the painful vertebra and apply oscillation. I have no comment or experience in this type of manipulation.

Acupuncture

This Chinese science being practiced for more than two thousand years believes that there are flowing energy channels around the human body, running through the so-called acupuncture meridians. Disruption of this pattern of energy flow may result in pain. A stimulation of a specific meridian will restore the energy flow called chi, ki or qi. Acting in "accupoints" (there are several hundred of accupoints distributed along the meridians which effect a specific organ) stimulates the meridian system that will bring relief of pain by "rebalancing" yin, yang, and qi. (or chi or ki). Accupoints are usually located by palpation, similar to trigger points. Penetrating the skin with a specific needle, which is twirled rapidly and intermittently for few minutes performs stimulation of the meridian system. There is a modification of this treatment (a money maker) by using low electrical current applied to the accupoints. (I do not recommend it.)

The mechanism of action could be the stimulation of endorphin production, generating analgesia (absence of pain) and perhaps an anti-inflammatory effect (endorphin is like an endogenous opium compound, produced by your own body, pituitary and hypothalamus in the brain, resembling somehow opiates, producing sense of well-being).

Acupuncture was introduced in USA around 1970. I attended an acupuncture symposium in Tokyo, many years ago, and I remember we were told the importance of the angle of contact between the needle and the skin and specially the thickness of the silver needle, a "thin one" will bring "energy charge," a "thick one" will bring "energy discharge" (believe it or not).

I previously stated that in my experience, I saw many patients who got relief of chronic low back pain by undergoing acupuncture. Done by a professional, it is an innocuous treatment, and I see no reason for not trying it.

Reiki

A new treatment imported from Japan. It seems to be a healing technique originated in Tibet over 2,500 years ago. It claims universal life force energy healing through direct application of Chi. It is believed that Reiki can relieve low back pain, boosting the immune system mainly when often linked to emotional, mental, and spiritual well-being. In this energy healing technique, the practitioner can channel the Reiki energy from the universe to his hands and transmit it to the patient's body, which will heal itself.

I just mention this new technique so the reader knows I keep up with my reading. If anybody tries, please let me know. I do not believe or recommend it.

Pilates

Joseph Pilates developed in the early twentieth century this physical fitness system. His method seems to believe that the mind control the muscular system, emphasizes breathing and exercises for the alignment of the spine. Strengthening and stretching of the dorsolumbar muscles. Breathing and mental concentration are part of this physical fitness system. I have no experience with Pilates.

Epidural Injection

It has to be done by an experienced anesthesiologist. A spinal needle is inserted into the epidural space, with the same technique used for the epidural block I already explained, using a combination of an anesthetic with a steroid. I do recommend it for those cases of low back pain not relieved by more conservative measures. In my experience, it is a very acceptable type of treatment; I have seen it work in lumbosacral radiculitis and spinal stenosis cases, saving the patient a surgical procedure.

Epidural perineural injections with autologous conditioned serum (ACS)—It is a recent method using a similar technique to the abovementioned epidural injection, substituting the steroid solution with autologous conditioned serum (ACS, Orthokine, which is enriched with interleukin-1, which seem to play a role in the cause [pathophysiology] of low back pain).

According to Becker and collaborators it is "potentially superior to steroid injection" (Efficacy of epidural perineural injections with autologous conditioned serum for radicular lumbar compression: an investigator-initiated, prospective, double blind, reference-controlled study. Spine. 2007; 32(17): 1803-8. University of Bochum, Germany).

Facet Injection

Injection of a local anesthetic combined with a steroid, usually guided under fluoroscopy to find the facet.

In my opinion this method just blocks the nerve supply of the facets. I have no experience on this treatment, and I can only state that when doing open surgery it is almost impossible to visualize the facet joint without removing bone, in other words the procedure works like a block of the surrounding facet (peri-joint block), but not going to the facet joint itself; however, the importance is that many patients have relief of pain with this method; why not try then?

I have the same comment for the use of radio frequency for denervation of the facet joints in the treatment of low back pain.

Trigger Point Injections

I have already discussed the subject. These are extremely tiny pinpoint painful areas, founded by finger touch over the low back region; anatomically speaking, they are located over the myofascial region (muscles and the thin flat tissue that covers them, called capsule).

According to Hachett, "trigger point pain is an area of hypersensitive somatic sensory nerve receptors that respond more readily and with increased intensity to stimuli of pressure and tension. (Ligament and Tendon Relaxation Treated by Prolotherapy, George S. Hackett, MD, third edition, C Thomas)

There are many theories that explain how the injection of the trigger points with an anesthetic combined with a steroid relieves back pain, but they do. They help and don't harm.

I would like to add that many patients may have tender and painful to palpation, small like "marbles" (fibrolipomas) benign tumors, made of fibrous and fat tissue over the low back region. Frequently, I would inject them with the previous combination and this would be followed by complete remission of symptoms.

Prolotherapy

From the word *proli* (Latin) meaning offspring; *proliferate*—to produce new cells in rapid succession (*Webster's Dictionary*). Hackett defines prolotherapy as applied medically in the treatment of skeletal disability; it is the rehabilitation of an incompetent structure by the generation of a new cellular tissue" (Ligament and Tendon Relaxation Treated by Prolotherapy, George S. Hackett, MD, third edition, C Thomas).

"According to Hackett, skeletal disability is due to ligament 'relaxation'; the strength of the ligament fibers has become impaired so that stretching of the fibrous strands occurs when the ligament is submitted to normal or less than normal tension and causes low back pain. So prolotherapy is the treatment of relaxed ligaments by the injection of a sclerosing agent into the ligaments and tendons. This injection sets-up a proliferative reaction which follows the laws of 'inflammation,' the end result of which is the formation of fibrous connective tissue" (A Myers MD, Bulletin of Hospital for J. Diseases Vol. xxii #1 April 1961); in other words, the growth of a very strong tendon.

Prolotherapy was popular in the fifties and sixties. It's mentor was Dr. Hackett. In his original article provided by the Prolotherapy Association, Prolotherapy for Sciatica from Weak Pelvic Ligaments and Bone Dystrophy "recommends it to alleviate low back pain, including sciatica."

I was lucky to have known, in Philadelphia, Dr. A. Myers, an orthopedic surgeon who had great experience with prolotherapy. He treated patients from the whole Delaware Valley and neighboring states. Dr. Myers showed me his technique and the preparation of the sclerosing solution. The solution used to contain dextrose, phenol, and glycerin, but later on he modified it to just dextrose and a local anesthetic. I saw many patients of Dr. Myers with excellent results. I am not aware of how many orthopedic surgeons or physical medicine physicians do perform prolotherapy today. I refer you to the American Prolotherapy Association (see useful resources chapter).

The current theory of low back pain points out to the joints (discs and facets) like the cause of the problem and not to the ligaments.

Chapter 10

My Exercise Program

Goal: To Increase Endurance/Strength of Abdominal Extensor Muscles

You should have in mind that in each exercise you should stop when you reach a painful range of motion.

First Group (fig. 32)

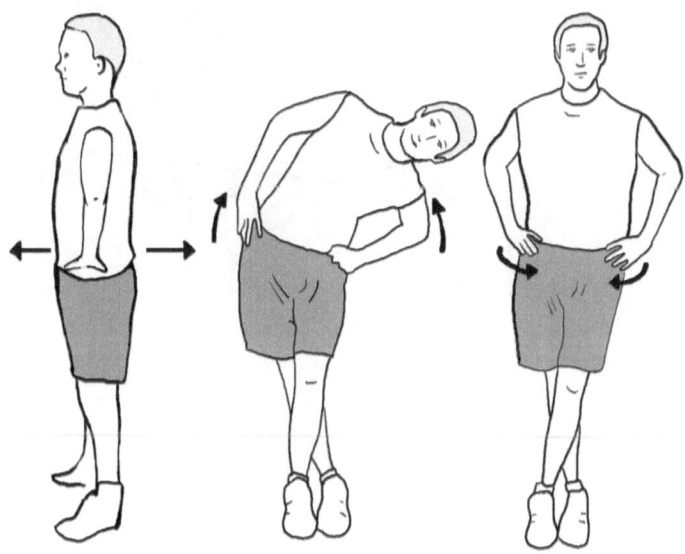

Fig. 32

In standing position, with a one-foot separation between the legs, do the following:

Flex (bend forward) slowly your trunk like trying to touch your toes with your fingers. When you reach maximum range, hold and count slowly to ten (seeking endurance). Repeat eight times.

Extension: Bend backward as much as possible and stop when pain appears, hold and count to ten. Repeat eight times.

Lateral bending to right and left with arms at your side. Bend first to right followed by left bend. Hold and count to ten. Repeat eight times each side.

Trunk rotation: to right and left with hands and forearms touching your breast. Hold and count to ten. Repeat eight times.

Second Group: Sitting (fig.33)

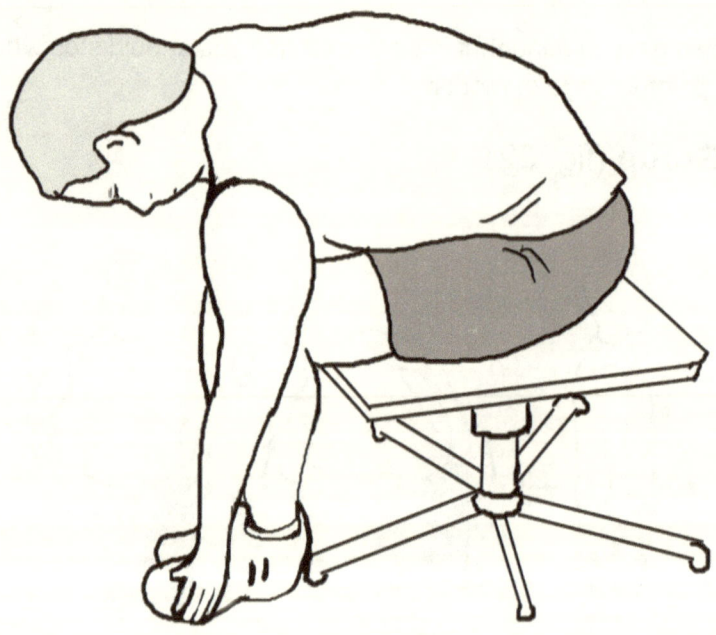

Fig. 33

Sitting on a stool or hard chair, bend forward trying to touch or grasp your ankles with your hands. Hold and count to ten. Repeat eight times.

Third Group: Lie on the floor over a mat

1. Abdominal (simple)

    Lie in supine position (face up) with your thighs flexed (knees bent at ninety degrees)(fig. 35). Place your hands in a resting position behind your neck. From this position slowly raise your upper trunk or shoulders from the floor about ten inches or twenty-five centimeters. Hold and count to ten. Repeat slowly eight times.

2. Abdominal with rotation of lumbar spine

    Same position as the previous exercise, while elevating your trunk, twist to the right while the left elbow is pointing to your right knee, now return to the floor and start twisting to the left while right elbow points to left knee (fig.36). Hold and count to ten. Repeat slowly eight times each.

3. Lumbar spine extension

    Lie in prone position (face down) on the floor as before. Stay flat on your chest, abdomen, and legs; rest your hands and forearms in your lower mandible. Now lift your chest from the floor as much as you can, few inches, about ten centimeters, hold and count to ten (endurance), return to horizontal or starting position. Repeat eight times (fig. 34 and 37).

    Make time to get involved in some activity like walking, jogging, swimming, or bicycling.

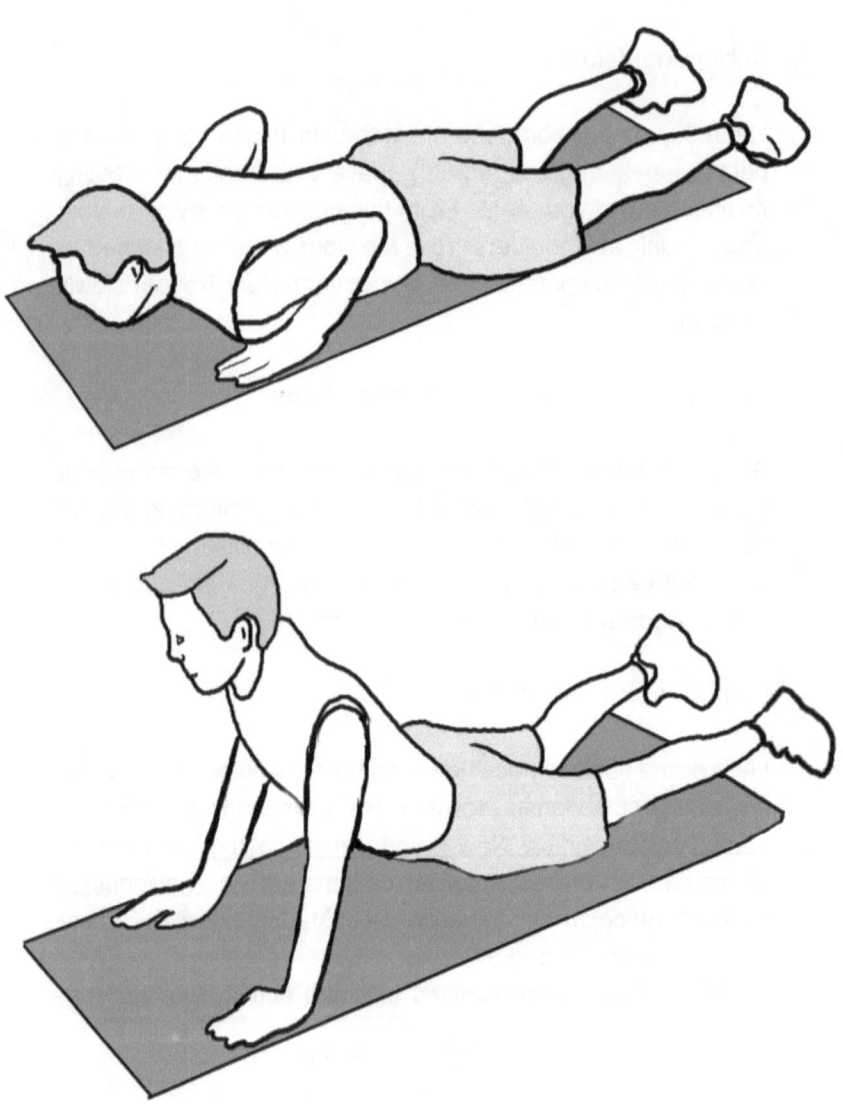

Fig. 34

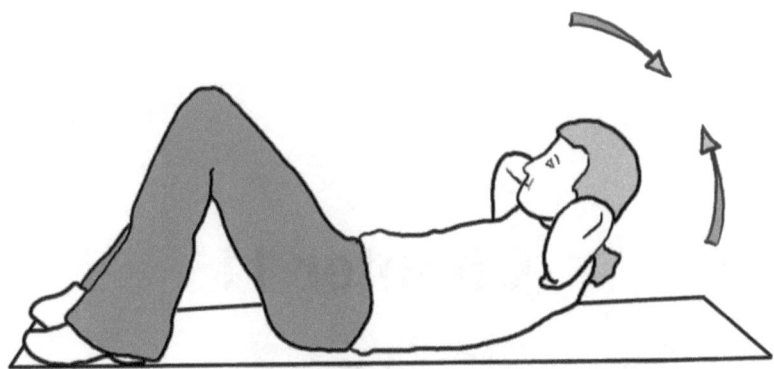

Supine Flexed Knees

Fig. 35

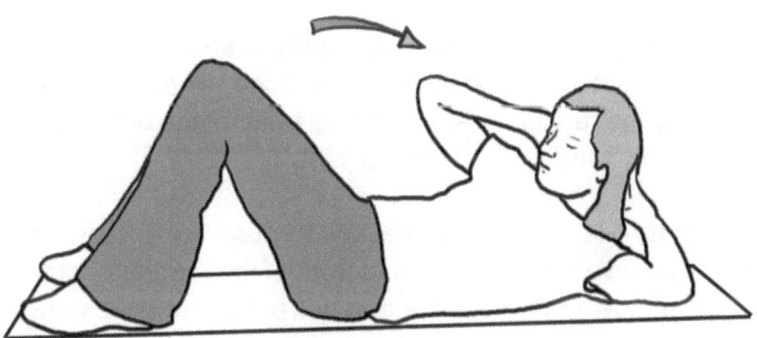

Abdominal with Rotation

Fig. 36

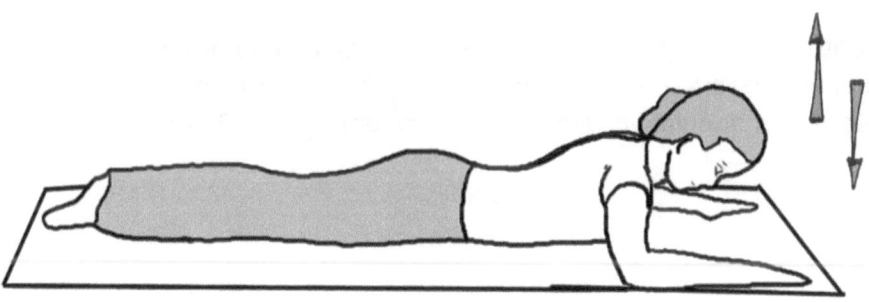

Prono Lift Chest

Fig. 37

Chapter 11

Posture and Ergonomics

Posture. According to Taber's Cyclopedic Medical Dictionary (ninth edition) "is an attitude or position of the body." Practically, posture is determined by the relation of "the line of gravity" of the entire spine to the "center of gravity" and "axis of the hip joint."

Line of gravity—is a line which passes through the center of the skull (second cervical vertebra), passes in front of the "center of gravity" and upper sacrum down the hip joints and in front of the knees and ankles joints.

Hip axis—line which passes from the center of the hip joint all the way down in front of the knee and ankle joints.

Center of gravity—as previously stated, is located around the second lumbar vertebra in the upright position, the pelvis is in about thirty-five degrees of angulation with the spinal column (figs. 38, 39).

Center of Gravity
Axis of Hip Joint

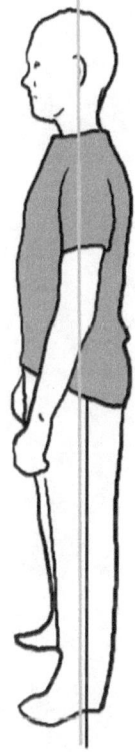 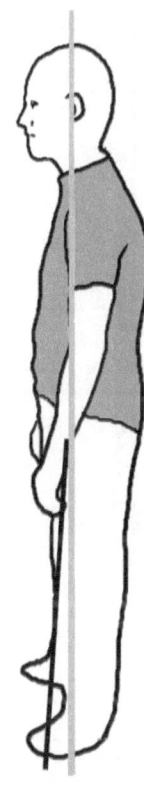 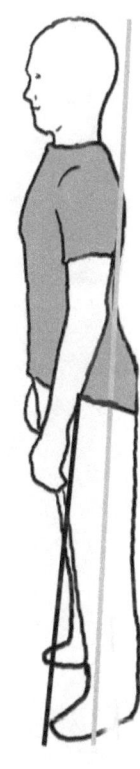

| Normal Posture
Center of Gravity
and Axis of Hip in Line | Relaxed Posture
Slightly Backward
Center of Gravity
falls behind joint axis | Military Posture
Center of Gravity falls
forward Abdomin drawn in |

Fig. 38

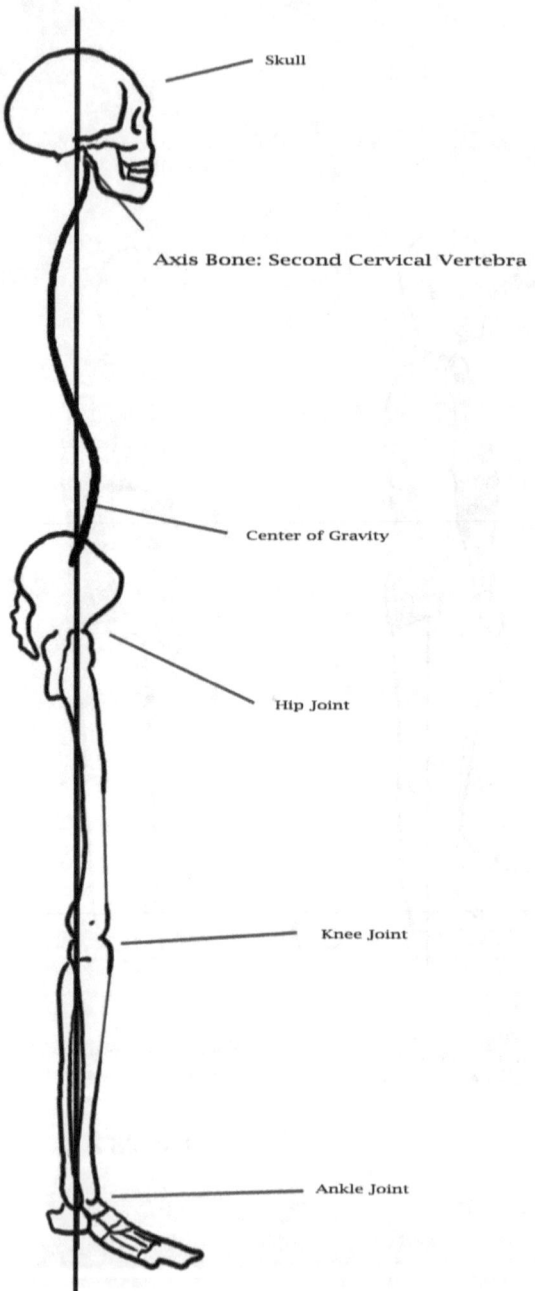

Fig. 39

Braune and Fisher, according with Steindler Kinesiology, described three types of posture (figs. 38, 39), namely:

1. Normal posture—Center of gravity and the line of gravity stand vertically over the common hip joint axis.
2. Relaxed posture—The body is slightly backward; the line of gravity and the center of gravity falls behind the axis of the hip joint.
3. Military posture—The thorax is forward, the abdomen is drawn-in, the line of gravity is backward, the axis of the hip joint and the center of gravity falls forward.

A correct posture, according to Mc Kenzie, is important to prevent low back pain, especially for those people who must stand for prolonged period of time.

"The body should be comfortable, usually in this position the chest will sag, the abdomen will protrude, and the lumbar spine will adopt extreme lordosis" (backward concavity).

"To acquire a good posture you should stand as tall as you can; you should lift your chest up; you should pull your stomach in and tighten your buttocks."

When keeping this posture you will reduce your lordosis (backward concavity).

Pathological or abnormal posture occurs when there is a discrepancy between the spine and the line of gravity like you see in those persons called "flat back;" they have an almost straight dorsal spine instead of a normal khyphosis (backward convexity), marked increase of the normal lumbar lordosis (backward concavity), and a protruded abdomen with fall of the abdominal organs.

I will now mention some common examples of wrong posture:

Nursing mothers. They usually sit with many pillows behind the dorsal region (thorax) with no support over the lumbar region, so the spine seeing from the side shows a dorsolumbar khyphosis (long curve with backward convexity). A large and hard pillow should be placed instead in the lumbar region to produce a lumbar lordosis (backward concavity).

Sitting: A person should sit straight up, to avoid a dorsolumbar khyphosis, he/she should seat forming a lumbar lordosis (see explanation in above paragraph).

   Posture in bed: when sitting, place a pillow behind the lumbar region to accomplish lordosis and avoid khyphosis. The best is to sleep in bed lying in lateral or side position. The best position to read is the prone one (flat on your stomach) and with the book or paper on the floor.

   Some people do still scrub floors. Be sure you do it with the hips flexed at ninety degrees, putting weights on your knees (lordosis), not with your legs under your thighs, showing khyphosis (fig. 40).

Scrubbing the Floor

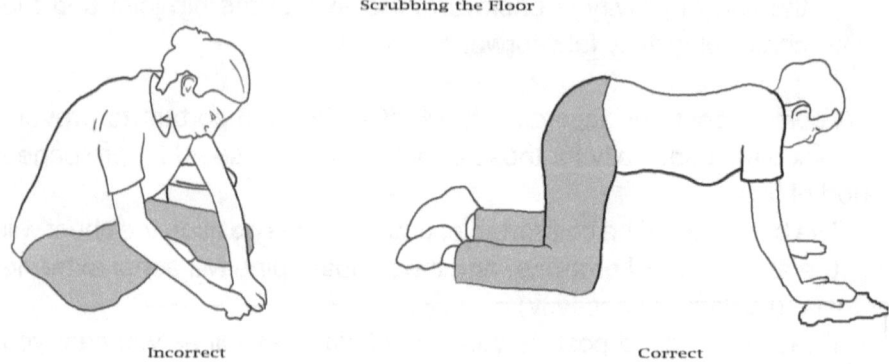

Incorrect   Correct

Fig. 40

   Lifting—protect your back while lifting from the ground, bend your knees.

   Sit—don't stand when working on a desk. Otherwise lift the desk or table to almost chest level to avoid a "bending" position (khyphosis).

   Finally, avoid slouching when traveling in a car, train, or airplane, or sitting at home, as it's so common in adolescents. You have to maintain a lordosis. (fig. 41)

Sitting on a Chair

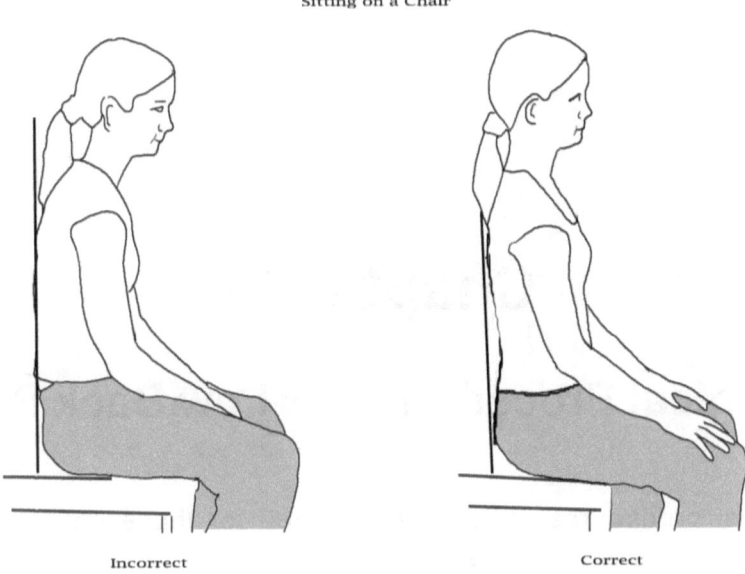

Incorrect   Correct

Fig. 41

Well, at this time you may be tired of reading lordosis and khyphosis, so I put the case to rest.

Fortunately, in the last few decades, a new science called ergonomics (from the Greek word *ergon)* which is most often translated to as function, task, or work has surged, dealing with the design of instruments and their applications for the comfort and safety of the workers, especially to prevent back injuries, muscles strains, tendons ruptures, falls, fractured bones, burns, eye troubles, etc. It proved to be useful in the prevention of low back pain.

Chapter 12

Surgical Procedures for Low Back Pain

Surgical procedures should be reserved for those cases where "conservative" treatment has failed.

Previously, I have stated that in my opinion no more than 5% of all cases fall into this category.

Again I would like to emphasize once more the following:

1. The importance of having a second or third opinion.
2. The need to investigate the surgical experience of the surgeon.
3. Bear in mind that patients with psychological problems or "secondary gains" (workmen's compensation) may have a different prognosis and recovery of any surgical intervention.

The purpose of this chapter is to familiarize the reader with past or present surgical procedures, in other words a practical explanation of the most known operations.

Chemonucleolysis

A procedure, popular, in the sixties and seventies, for the treatment of a herniated lumbar disc.

An enzyme (like meat tenderizer), obtained from the fruit of *Carica papaya*, by a special "surgical technique" is injected into the intervertebral disc; this enzyme, like digestion, quickly dissolves the nucleus pulposus.

The enzyme only attacks or destroys the disc without harming the bone or ligaments.

The procedure did dissolve the disc, but many dangerous complications did occur, even mortality. It obviously was discontinued.

Thermal Therapies

1. Thermal annulplasty is the application of heat, radio frequency, laser, or cold (cryoablation). These modalities are preformed with a coil over the periphery of the disc (annulus), and the disc tissue (discal collagen) shrinks, and produces a so-called denervation (kills the nerves) so the pain goes away. The general opinion is that these techniques are ineffective.
2. Facet neurotomy is another procedure that uses a catheter or an electrode to cut or cauterize the tiny nerves that innervates the facets with the purpose of relieving the pain. My opinion is this type of treatment is ineffective.

Lumbar Laminectomy

Laminectomy, total or partial (hemilaminectomy, right or left), is the removal of the laminae of the vertebrae (ectomy=removing) to gain access to the nerve roots, spinal cord, herniated lumbar discs or to decompress the spinal canal like what is done for spinal stenosis (fig. 42).

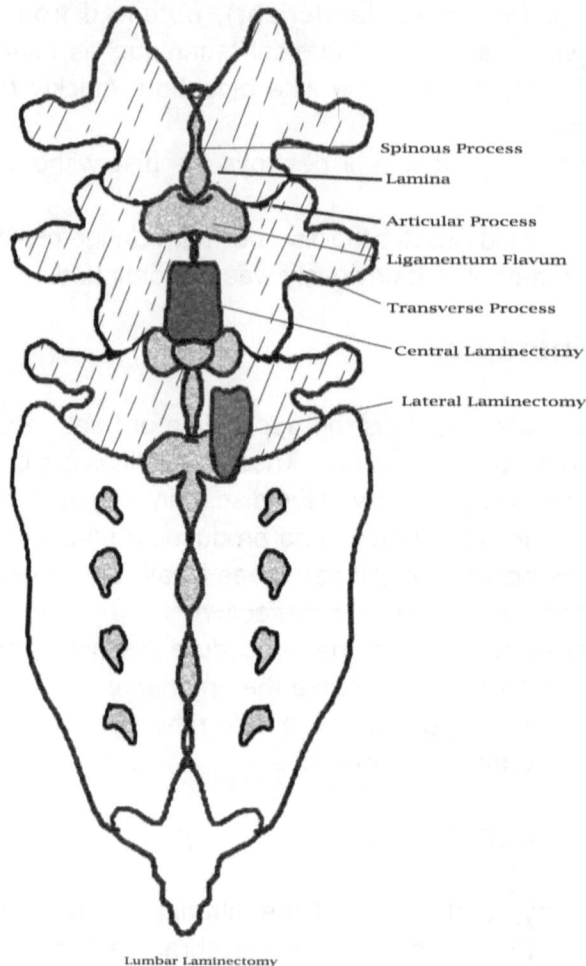

Lumbar Laminectomy

Fig. 42

The procedure can be performed under direct visualization or with the microscope (minimal invasive technique). It is the most common intervention done by neurosurgeons or orthopedic surgeons. It is an adequate and excellent procedure, rapid postoperative recovery, when properly indicated.

Arthrodesis of the Spine or Spinal Fusion

Spinal fusion (arthrodesis) is a surgical procedure with the objective of making rigid the damaged area of the spine. The abnormal or unstable motion between the vertebrae; due to mechanical disc or facet degeneration (the cause of low back pain) is alleviated by this accomplished rigidity, providing pain relief.

The fusion is accomplished by bridging two or three vertebrae with a bone graft. The bone graft could be "autogenous," meaning bone from the same patient, like the pelvis bone, or an "allograft," meaning bone from a donor like a cadaver (fig. 43).

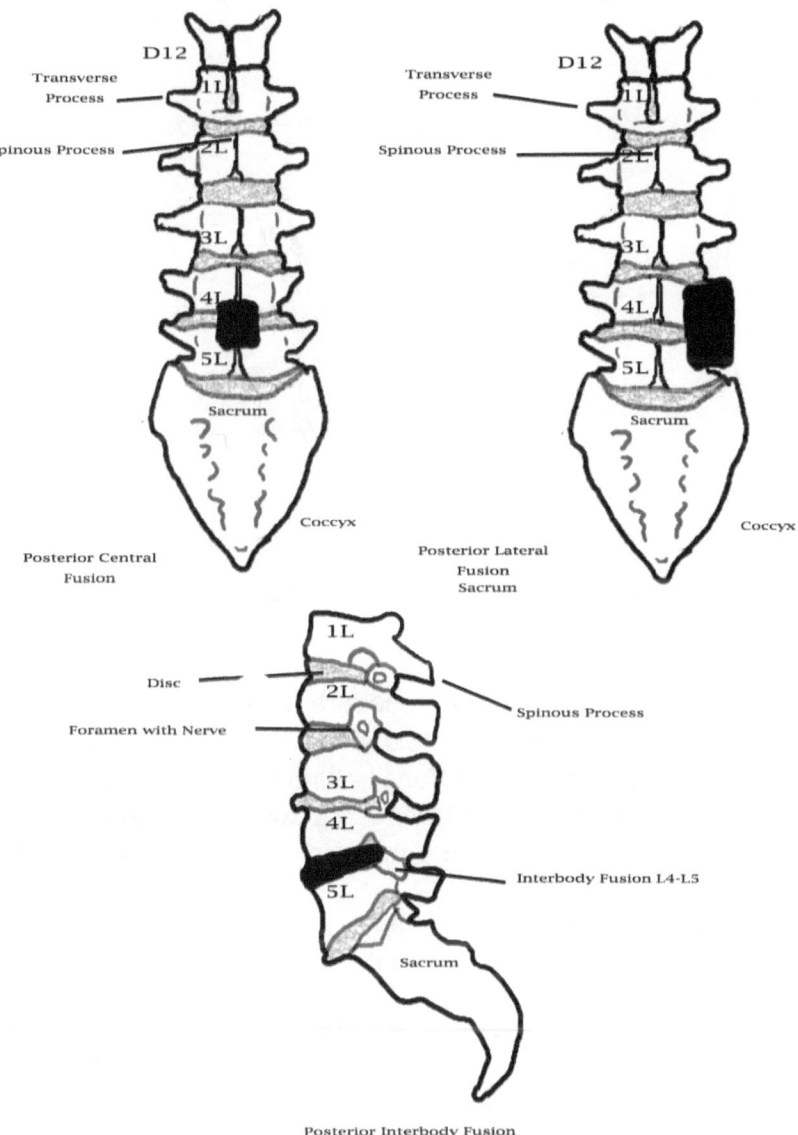

Fig. 43

The goal of the operation is that in a short period of time, this bone will be incorporated to the vertebrae forming a solid rigid mass. Sometimes, due to different causes the graft will not attach ("unite") to the vertebrae, with resulting motion. To avoid this nonunion, the fusion is reinforced with some hardware-like metal plates—pedicle screws and facet screws—made out of a material like titanium or stainless steel, which usually will not produce a foreign body reaction (fig. 44).

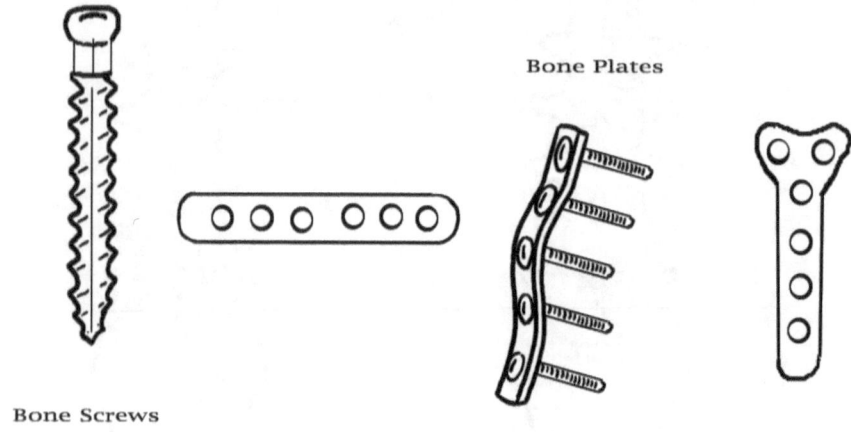

Fig. 44

The arthrodesis or fusion according to location of the graft could be classified as follows:

1. Anterior approach—The procedure is performed from the front of the vertebrae, through the abdomen, retro—or transperitoneal (the surgical approach is done behind the peritoneum or through it). This procedure could cause visceral or vascular injuries which could harm the presacral nerve plexus, which control ejaculation.
2. Posterior approach (the most commonly used)—The procedure is performed from the back of the spine and could be:

   a. Postero-lateral—Meaning lateral to the spinous process right and left side.
   b. Posterior interbody fusion—According to the location of the graft, could be lateral or transforaminal. Dr. R. B. Cloward, from Hawaii, made this procedure popular around 1953. (The

treatment of ruptured lumbar intervertebral discs by vertebral body fusion. Journal of Neurosurgery 1953; 10: 154-168). Using a posterior approach (from the back), the herniated or degenerated disc is excised, and the intervertebral space is grafted with a bone graft so both vertebral bodies will grow together and, as a result, motion at that level will be abolished. Sometimes the procedure could be reinforced by pedicles or facet screws, (two; figs. 45, 46).

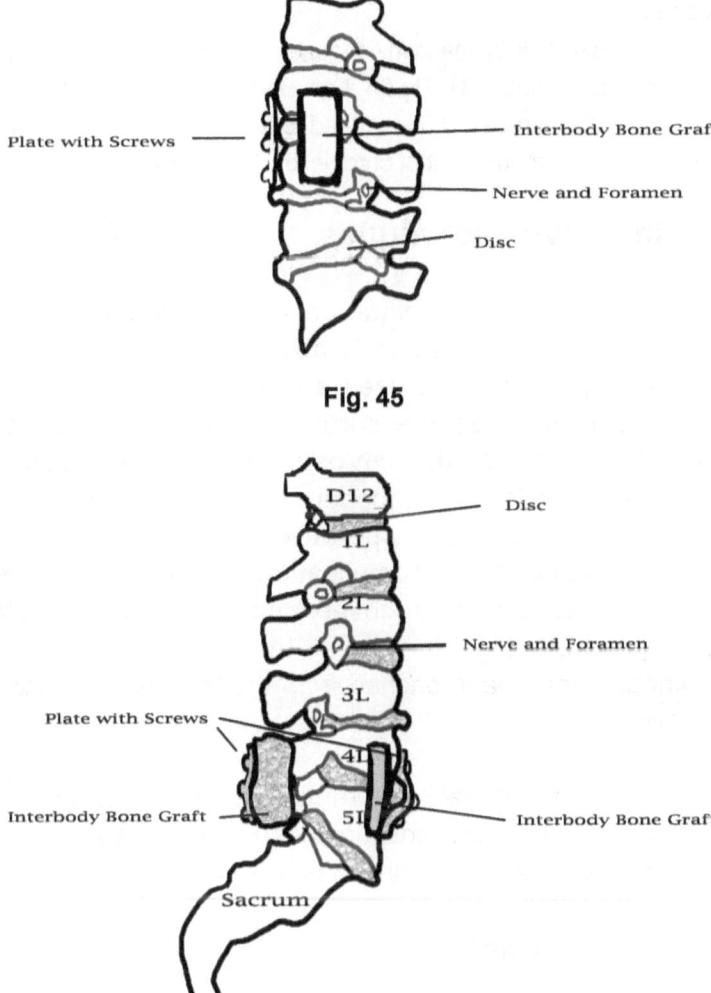

Fig. 45

Fig. 46

c. Posterior-anterior fusion or circumferential—The spine is fused in front and also behind with bone grafts, with plating or pedicle or facet screws for better immobilization (fig. 46).

d. Lateral fusion—called "Ozgur spine," is an extreme, very lateral interbody fusion (Ozgur Spine 2006 Jul-Aug; 6[4] 435-43).

Arthrodesis or fusion of segments of the spine, are well accepted surgical procedures, its indications and results depends of what condition or disease is being treated (like after resection of a bone tumor).

According to the American Academy of Orthopaedic Surgeons (monograph series # 31, Pg 64, Low Back Pain, Ed L.G. Jenis, MD), "additional research is required to further define the role of fusion in the management of chronic low back pain."

Minimal Invasive Techniques

This recent and new technique has been introduced to general surgery and now being used in lumbar spine surgery. Similar to an abdominal laparoscopy, it uses a tube with a lens from where the surgeon can visualize the surgical field and introduce small instruments to accomplish the extirpation or removal of soft or hard tissues. By definition, these procedures are less traumatic, making tiny surgical cuts, taking less operative time, the wounds healing faster with less incidences of complications like infections, bleeding, etc. Patients do have a faster recovery and are able to return to work in a shorter period.

The lumbar spine is approached from the front or the back, in the following manner:

1. In the anterior approach, the removal of the disc is done through the abdominal cavity (transperitoneal). It is a relatively dangerous method because there are mayor vessels and nerves in the way.

2. In the posterior approach we have:

   a. Percutaneous nucleotomy and nucleoplasty—Under local anesthesia and fluoroscopy control, a decompression of the nucleus of the disc is performed. The procedure is accomplished by using a motorized probe, which partially removes part of the disc. Other techniques instead use a laser ray to vaporize the disc material.

b. Percutaneus posterolateral lumbar disectomy and decompression—Performed under fluoroscopy, creating a small incision using a tiny cannula and a modified arthroscope (a working tube with lens to magnify the area). The surgeon makes a small hemilaminectomy (only one side of the laminae, right or left) and removes the herniated disc. (Shaffer J L, Kambin P., J BJS 73-A, 822-831,1991)

3. There are other techniques using also a tiny incision where after the hemi-laminectomy, they place a bone graft (fusion) reinforced with pedicles screws in the area.

Dynamic Stabilization Devices

A way to stabilize an area (segment) of disc degeneration without performing a spinal fusion (arthrodesis), where contrary to a fusion, the motion of the treated area is maintained, it is an operation that prevents mainly abnormal motion and perhaps contributes to a "self"-disc repair. The procedure is carried out from the back (posterior).

1. Pedicle screw dynamic systems—are synthetic flexible ligaments attached to vertebral bone by way of pedicle screws, like the Dynesys device. The Diam is a polyester-encased silicone dynamic stabilization device. (Jean Taylor, MD; Patrick Pulpin, MD; Stephanie Delajoux MD; Sylvia Palmer, MD. 5/10/2007 Neurosurgical Focus 2007, 22(1) 2007. American Academy of Neurological Surgeons). This procedure is being done; in my opinion more data is required.

2. Interspinous Spacers—are devices which produce distraction or separation between two vertebrae, giving more room to the spinal cord and nerve roots, mainly indicated for the treatment of spinal stenosis; most of the data were coming from Europe. The most known is the X-Stop, a titanic implant. The X-Stop reduces extension of the spinal segment, preventing narrowing

of the spinal canal while preserving motion in flexion, lateral bending, and rotation. (Neurosurgery Focus 2007,22 (1) C 2007AmAss of N. Surgeons). Precise selection or indication is necessary; not every patient with spinal stenosis is a good candidate for this relative simple procedure. (Appropriate Selection of Patients with lumbar spinal stenosis for interspinous Process Decompression with the X-Stop by Carl Lauryssen, MD. California, Beverly Hills.). It is also my opinion that this procedure has an excellent future.

Facet Arthroplasty

It is a procedure where the degenerated (arthritic) facet joint, two in each vertebra, is replaced by an allergic material. According to Richard Guyer, MD (Motion Preservation Technologies and their outcome, Symposia Spine, Proceeding 2007 Annual meeting of the American Academy of Orthopaedic Surgeons) there are several undergoing clinical evaluation, these are pedicle screw based implants.

Disc Replacement or Disc Arthroplasty

Total disc replacement is a substitution of the annulus fibrosus and nucleus pulposus of the damaged disc. The goal is to retain or obtain joint function, meaning motion and high loading capacity of the disc in the lumbar region.

Several devices with low friction and sliding surface have been designed, some made of metal or plastic articulating surface to contact the above and below vertebrae (fig. 47). Most of these devices are implanted through an anterior approach (abdomen), which is a more difficult procedure.

Disc Arthroplasty

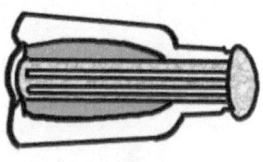

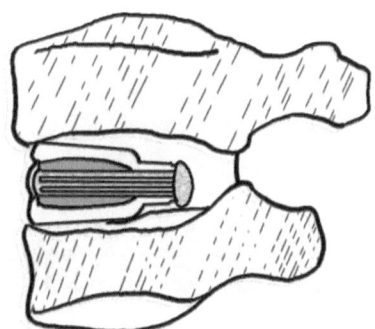

Lumbar Disc
Prosthesis

Prosthesis Replacing
Lumbar Disc

Fig. 47

These procedures are still somewhat experimental ("The result of Disc Arthroplasty are not known for long term studies, Pg. 285 "Proceding" Feb14-18 2007 of the American Academy of Orthopaedic Surgeons 2007 Annual Meeting).

Chapter 13

Painkillers or Analgesics

I like now to say few words about analgesics or painkillers.

First let me explain with this small "story," about in general, what you should know about a drug or medicament.

While traveling around the world, gathering with tourists like myself, sooner or later people want to know what you do. Well, as soon they realize I am a physician, well I cannot escape the medical questions.

Mrs. Martinez asked, "Doc, what do you think of Dioxaflex Forte for pain?"

I answered, "Mrs. Martinez, I really do not know about that painkiller, I am not familiar with that name." Well, you should have seen how she looked at me! I am sure she thought, "What kind of a doctor is this guy?"

I said, "Mrs. Martinez, I may be able to help you if I am able to see the chemical formula of this drug." She brought the little bottle with the pills. I read this medication was a tablet; the drug was a compound of diclofenac sodico and codeine. So I gave her my medical opinion about the combination of an NSAID (nonsteroidal anti-inflammatory drug) and codeine, an opiate.

I told this story to point out that the reader should be aware there are a limited number of drugs with analgesic properties, perhaps no more than fifty. Pharmaceutical laboratories give them different names, marketing them like a new "miracle medicament" (when the composition may be just an aspirin with an enteric coat).

I want to warn you to be aware that the trademark does not mean much; the real McCoy is the chemical formula of the drug.

A painkiller, like any medicine, has its specific action, like to decreasing, alleviating, or taking pain away. They also may have side effects to some organs like liver and kidney (main detoxification of the body); they may be contraindicated with some medical conditions, may have adverse reactions, could have a negative INTERACTION with another drug that you are taking; the patient could be allergic to such drug; and finally, it could create dependence and withdrawal reaction, mainly when using opiates.

I classified analgesics or painkillers, according to the magnitude of pain, as follows:

mild, moderate, or severe pain.

Mild Pain

For mild pain, I advise the intake of acetaminophen (like Tylenol), aspirin (ASA), and nonsteroidal anti-inflammatory drugs (NSAID).

Acetaminophen (Tylenol, the trademark most known in this country; Panadol; Lemogrip; Napa; and Tempra) is an excellent analgesic.

ASA and NSAIDs—they are painkillers and antypiretic (lowers body temperature), anti-inflammatory, and they have somewhat a platelet-inhibitory action (like a blood thinner drug).

These medications should be taken with precautions; they are irritants of the stomach and intestine lining and could cause an ulcer or gastrointestinal bleeding. An ulcer complication is a perforation and peritonitis (severe infection of the abdominal cavity, with high mortality).

Except aspirin, they can increase the chance of a heart attack and a stroke. Aspirin, however, could cause bleeding in the brain, stomach, and intestines beside ulcers.

Finally, the reader should be aware of kidney and liver toxicity when abused.

Acetaminophen (like Tylenol) is extremely dangerous with the intake of alcohol because it is capable of causing an acute and mortal liver failure.

Few words about NSAIDs, COX-2 inhibitors, which do not harm your stomach or intestines—celecoxib (trademark Celebrex). FDA took another

COX-2 out of the market because of possible production of a heart attack (acute myocardial infarction) Viox.

A physician should prescribe COX-2 inhibitors.

Many of these drugs are available over the counter, no prescription necessary; however, they sell with smaller dose, making the therapeutic value somewhat questionable, so you may have to double the medication.

Summing-up, serious side effects include:

1. Heart attack
2. Stroke
3. High blood pressure
4. Heart failure from water retention
5. Kidney condition, danger of failure
6. Bleeding and ulcers in stomach or bowels
7. Anemia (less red cells)
8. Skin reactions
9. Allergic reactions
10. Liver problems to failure
11. Asthma attacks in people with asthma

Acetylsalicylic Acid or Aspirin or ASA

    Aspirin (Bayer and others)
    Alka-Seltzer
    Anacin
    Ascriptin
    Bufferin
    Ecotrin

List of Nonsteroidal Anti-inflammatory Drugs (NSAIDs)

Generic Name	Trademark
Ibuprofen	Motrin, Advil
Naproxen sodium	Aleve, Anaprox
Naproxen	Naprosyn
Ketoprolen	Actron

Choline magnesium trisalicylate	Trilisate
Ketoprofen	Orudis
Diflunisal	Dolobid
Etodolac	Lodine
Celecoxib	Celebrex
Diclofenac	Cataflan, Voltaren, Arthrotec (with misoprostol)
Fenoprofen	Nalfon
Flurbiprofen	Ansaid
Indomethacin	Indocin, indameth
Ketoprofen	Oruvail, Orudis
Mefenamic acid	Penstel
Meloxicam	Mobic
Nabumetone	Relafen
Oxaprozin	Daypro
Piroxicam	Feldene
Sulindac	Clinoril
Tolmetin	Tolectin
Meclofenamate	Meclomen

Misoprostol is a drug (like Cytotec) used to prevent NSAIDs-induced gastric ulcer in high-risk patients.

Moderate Pain

Propoxyphene	Darvon
Propoxyphene napsylate	Darvon-N
Propoxyphene napsylate, acetaminophen	Darvocet-N
Propoxyphene acetaminophen	Wygesic

Moderate to Severe Pain

Ketorolac (trademark Toradol)
It is used for short period of time (up to five days), mainly postoperative follow-up at home.

The patient was already with injectable Toradol while in the hospital. Usually given to patients, which require opioid level.

Severe Pain

Opioid analgesics are the treatment of choice for severe acute pain.

Short-term use is advised, dependence and addiction, contrary to some medical and public opinion, are extremely unlikely to develop. Physical dependence and/or tolerance may develop upon prolong use.

Elderly people are more sensitive to these painkillers, may experience greater peak effect, and longer duration of pain relief.

Patients taking these drugs should not do any of the following: use machinery, drive, or engage in any activity that could be dangerous since they may become dizzy or not be alert.

Codeine sulfate	Codeine
Hydromorphone	Dilaudid
Meperidine	Demerol
Morphine ext-rel	MS Contin
Oxycodone ext-rel	OxyContin
Oxycodone	OxyIR
Hydrocodone	Hydrocodone
Fentanyl transdermal	Duragesic
Tramadol	Ultram

Combination of any of the above drugs with acetaminophen (like Tylenol) or aspirin will increase the analgesic power.

Hydrocodone bitartrate, Acetaminophen	Vicodin, Norco, Lorcet
Oxycodone/Acetaminophen	Percocet, Tylox, Roxicet
Oxycodone with Aspirin	Percodan
Acetaminophen and Codeine phosphate	Tylenol, # 2/3/4
Hydrocodone bitartrate acetaminophen	Lorcet plus
Tramadol/acetaminophen	Ultracet
Hydrocodone/Ibuprofen	Vicoprofen
Dihydrocodeine, acetaminophen, and caffeine	DHC plus

Chapter 14

Useful Resources

American Academy of Orthopaedic Surgeons	*www.aaos.org*
American Association of Neurological Surgeons	*www.aans.org*
	www.neurosurgerytoday.org
American Board of Orthopaedic Surgery	*www.abos.org*
American College of Rheumatology	*www.reumathology.org/*
Annals of Internal Medicine	*www.annals.org/*
Arthritis Foundation	*www.arthritis.org*
	www.aana.org
Congress of Neurological Surgeons	*www.neurosurgeon.org/*
International Society of Arthroscopy, Knee Surgery and Orthopaedic Sports Medicine	*www.isakosonline.com*
Journal of the American Academy of Orthopaedic Surgeons	*www.jaaos.org*
Journal of the American College of Surgeons	*www.journalacs.org*
MD Linx	*www.mdlinx.com*
Medscape	*www.medscape.com*
Merkmedicus.com	*www.merkmedicus.com*
North American Spine Society	www.spine.org
The Journal of Bone & Joint Surgery	*www.ejbjs.org*
The Journal of the American Medical Association	htpp://jama.ama-assn.org
The Lancet Global Health Network	*www.thelancet.com*
The New England Journal of Medicine	*www.nejm.org*
US National Library of Medicine/National Institutes of Health	*www.nlm.nih.gov/*
Web Med	*www.webmed.com*

American College of Surgeons	*www.facs.org*
Archives of Surgery	*http://archsurg.ama-assn.org/*
American Orthopedic Society for Sport Medicine	*www.sportmed.org*
American Association of Orthopaedic Medicine	*www.aaomed.org/page*

Index

www.ingramcontent.com/pod-product-compliance
Lightning Source LLC
Chambersburg PA
CBHW031253280526
45784CB00004B/1838